What readers have said about *You*

"You and your book became my inspiration. I read the book over and over and over again – it helped to alleviate the overwhelming feeling of fear. Please don't ever underestimate the value of your book. You were my best friend through the whole experience." *Jacqui*

"During my third cycle of A/C I was at a very low point; I was in my bedroom crying when I decided to read your book again. After finishing I found the strength to get dressed, get in the car and go to the fruit shop. Even though I was very weak I managed it – your book gave me the strength to keep going." *Ros*

"I walked into the oncologist on Friday feeling very frightened about having to repeat my chemo/radiation treatment for recurring breast cancer and there was your book *You Can Get Through This*. What a great boost. I picked it up and felt your strong message within the first page. I read the rest as soon as I reached home and it has helped me to become strong and positive. I also loved the humour of your experiences that you put into the book, so you even had me laughing!!!" *Judith*

"You must read *You Can Get Through This*. I keep several copies ready for those times when friends of friends who have just been diagnosed contact me for direction and advice." *Lyn Swinburne AM,*
CEO Breast Cancer Network Australia

"My daughter read it after I did and it made a huge difference to both of us – she had a much better understanding of what I felt and what I was going through and I loved not having to try to explain. I'd recommend it to everyone who has a friend or family member with breast cancer."   *Jan*

"I enjoyed *You Can Get Through This* very much – I actually read it in one sitting. I couldn't put it down!"   *Julie*

"Domini's story is so real, so wonderful and so inspiring that I want other women to hear it. It's a great read for any woman, cancer or not."
Dr Rosie King MB, BS FACSHP
Author, broadcaster and public speaker

"Domini's book is filled with useful and practical advice to help women with breast cancer take control of their lives."   *Professor John Boyages*
Executive Director, NSW Breast Cancer Institute

"I found *You Can Get Through This* very inspirational and helpful."   *Annabel*

"A great book! I admired your strength for coping with it all on your own (with a sense of humour) and have drawn strength form it myself. I found the book most helpful and have it on the side table by my favourite chair for quick reference."   *Wendy*

"I found your book wonderful; you seemed to have an answer for all those questions I had asked myself."   *Lindy*

"It was just what I needed – an easy-to-read, down to earth account of what happens and how to cope with it all. It's a serious subject but Domini has managed to write with humour, making it the book an enjoyable as well as an informative read."   *Sue*

"Congratulations on your book – I thoroughly enjoyed reading it and it has helped me in lots of ways."   *Chris*

"Your book conveyed all the practical ways to live well, which is why I recommend it to anyone who contacts me for support and information."   *Annie*

You can get through this!

How to stay positive
when you're coping
with breast cancer

Domini Stuart

© Domini Stuart 2009

First edition published in 2001 by Domini Stuart

www.doministuart.com

Cover image: Tanya Dyhin
Cover design: Anmarie Dabinet

ISBN 0-97809579144-0-7

This book is intended to give general information only. The author does not dispense medical advice or prescribe, either directly or indirectly, any technique as a form of treatment for physical or medical problems without the advice of a physician. The author, publisher and distributors expressly disclaim all liability to any person arising directly or indirectly from the use of, or any errors or omissions in, the information in this book. The adoption and application of information in this book is at the reader's discretion and is his or her own responsibility.

For Lucas, Julius, Clio and Piers

With thanks to Amber St Clare, Danielle Walley, Anmarie Dabinet, Tanya Dyhin, Carissa Bolton and Annie Young, and to the many women who have shared their experiences and thoughts with me.

Domini Stuart was born in the midlands of England, studied human biology and psychology in London and moved to Sydney in 1982. She works as an advertising copywriter, freelance journalist and author; her latest book is *Staying Well After Breast Cancer – a gentle approach to taking care of the basics.*

CONTENTS

CHAPTER 14. WHEN THINGS GO WRONG   131
- No-one's life is perfect
- Fighting off depression
- Getting back in control

CHAPTER 15. YOU DON'T HAVE TO GET BACK TO NORMAL   135
- You may feel depressed when you stop your treatment
- Create a new 'normal' to move forward to
- Living with the fear

STAYING WELL AFTER BREAST CANCER   141

RECIPES   143

INDEX   157

INTRODUCTION
TO THE SECOND EDITION

When I was told I had breast cancer my life was already a mess. I felt helpless, overwhelmed and out of control; cancer seemed like the final straw.

It didn't help that I kept on hearing about needing to stay positive. I had been depressed for much of my adult life – how on earth could I start feeling positive now that I also had a double mastectomy, radiotherapy, two courses of chemotherapy and an uncertain future ahead of me?

It still amazes me that I did. Not in the spontaneous way that some people talk about – flowers didn't suddenly smell sweeter, nor did the rest of my problems simply cease to exist. Feeling more positive was something I learned to do.

The first step was understanding that I didn't have to pretend to be happy all the time, or that I never felt sad or afraid. Feeling positive was not a weighty responsibility – another burden I had to bear. It was about helping myself to feel better, as simple as that.

When I wrote the first edition of this book I was still in the final weeks of treatment and very eager to share all that I had learned. Nine years on, I still live my life by the same principles. New challenges inevitably arise and, when they do, I draw on the same strategies to help me to cope with them. For me, feeling more positive isn't just about cancer, it's about the quality of my everyday life.

1

YOU'VE FOUND A LUMP...

> - Every woman who finds a lump in her breast fears that she has breast cancer – and that she may not survive
> - It is vital to find out as quickly as possible whether or not your lump is breast cancer
> - Women who have never had a lump in their breast have no idea how you're feeling

If you find a lump in your breast it is very unlikely to be breast cancer. But if you have a lump in your breast right now, this fact is close to meaningless. As long as there is the slightest possibility that your lump *is* cancer you wouldn't be human if you didn't fear the worst. And only people who have been in your situation can truly understand the power of that fear.

Going to see your doctor takes courage. Some women put it off, hoping the lump is just a monthly 'hormonal thing' that will simply disappear. Others make the appointment before they finish getting dressed. However you react, when you're face to face with your GP, you are entitled to have your fears taken seriously. That means finding out as quickly as possible whether or not you have breast cancer.

In the first instance, this will mean having a mammogram and probably an ultrasound. If these tests are inconclusive, your doctor will probably recommend a fine needle biopsy, where a few of the suspicious cells are removed with a fine needle and sent to the lab for analysis. This is usually enough to confirm a positive or negative diagnosis and the results should be available the following day. In less usual cases, a more extensive biopsy may be needed involving a local or general anaesthetic.

All of these services are readily available in all but remote country areas. Even here it will be a question of how far you need to travel, not how long you need to wait.

If your doctor feels there is no need to hurry, he (I'm using he for convenience – a female doctor could be just as dismissive) must be made to understand how you feel. There may be no real urgency in a medical sense and your doctor knows that, statistically, your lump is unlikely to be cancer. But the reality is you probably feel as bad now as you will ever feel, whatever your test results. No doctor should prolong this torment for a moment longer than absolutely necessary.

If you don't feel strong enough to tackle an uncooperative doctor, take someone with you who does. If that's not possible, take this book and have him read the message for all GPs on the next page.

You may also have trouble with well-meaning friends. It's amazing how many 'know' that there's nothing to worry about. They may back up this 'knowledge' with experience – a cousin, an aunt and a neighbour who all found lumps just like yours that turned out to be nothing at all. The best thing you can do – preferably before your friends tell you to stop worrying – is thank them politely for their comments, then walk away before you feel a need to strangle them.

A message for all GPs

Every woman who comes to your surgery with a lump in her breast is afraid she's going to die.

You know that, statistically, the lump is unlikely to be cancer. You also know that, statistically, your patient is likely to survive even if it is. But statistics are totally irrelevant as long as breast cancer has the potential to kill anybody.

Your patient's fears are not groundless. She deserves to be treated with compassion and respect.

Most importantly, this means ensuring that she gets the fastest possible access to effective diagnostic procedures. This way, if she doesn't have cancer, her time of needless worry is reduced to the absolute minimum. If she does have cancer, she can get on with being treated.

Please don't make her wait a minute more than she has to. And never, ever tell her not to worry.

Perfect timing

I was unlucky enough to discover my lump on December 23rd. It was a week before I could see my GP, another week until the laboratories opened for a mammogram and ultrasound, and yet another week before I could have an appointment with my chosen surgeon.

The first plan was for me to wait until I saw my surgeon for the fine needle biopsy. But, like every other woman who has ever been told to wait, the uncertainty was ripping me apart.

I kept swinging wildly between the sickening fear that I might only have a short time to live and chiding myself for being a pessimistic drama queen. In my heart I knew that I had cancer, but I felt guilty if I started to think about what might happen next – as if I were willing bad news on myself.

The thought never left me for a moment. Everything that happened related back to cancer. I started to miss work deadlines because I simply couldn't concentrate and I agonised over what excuse to give my clients. Everyone who knew was telling me not to worry. That, of course, was like telling the sun not to rise.

Luckily, my GP was understanding. When I asked if I could have the biopsy done sooner she made an appointment with a local laboratory. Within a day diagnosis had been confirmed – and I felt strangely calm. Partly, no doubt, because I was in shock, but also because I now knew that I had breast cancer and could start preparing myself for what was going to happen next.

If you're about to have a fine needle biopsy...
According to women whose lumps were situated away from the nipple, this procedure is painless. However, if your lump is anywhere near your nipple, I strongly recommend that you ask for a local anaesthetic. Because my lump was quite solid, I needed three separate cell samples, each taken through the areola. The initial sting would have been a very worthwhile investment!

2

BREAST CANCER
IS NOT YOUR FAULT

- No-one knows what causes breast cancer
- You are not responsible for your breast cancer
- You don't have to feel guilty about any increased risk to your daughter
- Lumps sometimes get missed – it's not your fault

No-one knows what causes breast cancer. We know that certain faulty genes increase the risk of getting breast cancer, but not everyone who carries the fault will get the disease. Nor will every woman who had her first child after she was thirty, every woman who is stressed, keeps her emotions bottled up, drinks more than eight standard alcoholic drinks a week or has a poor diet.

All of these factors and many more besides may influence the development of breast cancer. With the right research, someone could probably present convincing evidence suggesting that women who listened to the Beatles are more likely to develop breast cancer.

My grandmother and my maternal aunt both had breast cancer when they were relatively young, which suggested there might be a genetic link. After my treatment I had a blood test which showed that I am, indeed, carrying a faulty BRCA2 gene. That still doesn't explain why I went on to develop cancer when others with the mutation don't.

> The doctor read out the result of the fine needle biopsy to a woman I know. It was positive. He then asked how old she was when she had her first child. When she told him 32 he raised his eyebrows and muttered 'Well, then...', as if breast cancer were the price she had to pay for not having her first baby in her teens or early twenties.
>
> Her first message about breast cancer was that it was her own fault. It wasn't.

Breast cancer is not a price you have to pay It could have been because I have, at various times of my life, drunk far too much, smoked like a chimney and lived on chocolate. It could have been because I had all four of my children in my thirties, or because I was nurturing some deep and unrecognised resentment. It could have been all or none of these things. It doesn't matter. There's nothing I can do to change my past. What matters is what I do now to manage my future.

Do you have a 'cancer personality'?

People who don't have cancer may take comfort in believing that they're different from people who do. One way of protecting themselves is to imagine that you have a 'cancer personality' – in other words, a personality that is totally different from their own.

You may have read descriptions of the cancer-prone person and you may even think it sounds a bit like you. But, unless you are you prepared to believe that every woman everywhere in the world who gets breast cancer has a personality identical to your own, you have to let go of the idea that you brought cancer on yourself by having the 'wrong' one.

Unless you took yourself into a laboratory and injected your breast with vast amounts of proven, tumour-inducing substances, there is no possible reason for you to feel responsible for your breast cancer.

There's no point in worrying about your past

When I was 21 I had an extremely cavalier attitude to my health. If someone had told me then that, unless I changed my ways, I would be diagnosed with breast cancer at the age of 47, I would have laughed at them. I'd have assumed there would be a cure by then – or that I'd either be dead already or too old to care.

Most of us wish we'd done at least some things differently when we were younger but we weren't the same people then. We can't blame ourselves for not being as sensible then as we are now.

You don't have to feel guilty about any increased risk to your daughter

One newly-diagnosed woman was told by her doctor 'You do know this makes it more likely that your daughter will get breast cancer, don't you?' This was not only unnecessarily cruel, it was very unlikely to be true.

Yes, if your daughter has inherited a genetic mutation from you she is statistically more likely to develop the disease. However, as only five per cent of all breast cancers appear to be due to a genetic malfunction, the chances of this happening are remote. Even if it were the case, not every woman who carries the gene will develop breast cancer. And it's hardly your choice – so there would absolutely no point in feeling guilty about it.

On the positive side, you will no doubt encourage your daughter to adopt the same, more optimistic outlook and healthier lifestyle that you are developing now. You will probably encourage regular screening. She may listen, she may not. You can't force good health on her. Painful as it can be to accept, there's only so much you can do to protect her, but that still doesn't make anything your fault.

When I discovered that I was carrying a BRCA2 mutation my daughter was 14 year old.

What I wanted to do was have her screened without telling her, find that she hadn't inherited the gene fault and breathe a big sigh of relief. Of course, there's no way a parent can have a child screened without his or her consent, and there's no way a child can give consent until he or she is 18. So I decided there was absolutely no point in raising the subject until then, if I raised it at all.

In the meantime, I did my best to discourage her from following the self-destructive behaviours once so beloved by her mother. I encouraged her to eat well, do some exercise and to avoid cigarettes.

By her 18th birthday I still wasn't sure that telling her was the right thing. I was worried that I might inadvertently plant the idea in her mind that breast cancer was inevitable for her, particularly as her great aunt died from the disease when she was only 22. But in the end I decided I didn't have the right to keep information from her that might in any way affect the choices she made, particularly in terms of screening.

I didn't choose to put her in a situation where she might have an increased chance of developing breast cancer. Whatever else I feel, I know there's no reason to feel guilty for that, and the same is true for you.

Lumps sometimes get missed – it's not your fault

If your cancer was no longer considered to be 'early' at the time of diagnosis, you may be blaming yourself for being less than vigilant. It's true that, when it comes to surviving breast cancer, early detection remains our most powerful ally. It's also true that no one method of detection is 100 per cent effective.

As I have a family history of breast cancer I had a mammogram every two years from the age of forty. I checked my breasts every day after the shower as I was applying moisturiser because the more familiar I was with the way they looked and felt, the more likely I was to pick up the smallest change. I also had a doctor examine my breasts each time I had a Pap test.

My very competent and thorough GP examined my breasts three weeks before I discovered a seven centimetre lump under one nipple. Later, my surgeon told me that it had probably been developing for around two years – yet I would swear that it appeared overnight.

My GP was horrified by the thought that she had missed a lump of that size but I don't for a minute think she did. It either couldn't be felt, or was indistinguishable from the normal, lumpy tissue in the other breast.

As far as mammograms were concerned, it was difficult to separate the lump from the surrounding, dense tissue even on the final diagnostic x-ray. While most lumps are not nearly so hard to find, it's hardly surprising that mine had been overlooked.

So, while I was concerned to discover that my cancer had spread into seven lymph nodes, I can accept that a tumour can remain undetected even after the most thorough routine screening.

Know what you're looking for

One thing that surprised me was the way my lump felt. I had always imagined that the thing I was hoping not to find would be spherical and distinct – like a pea under the skin. In fact mine was long and irregular, remarkably like normal glandular breast tissue.

I think it's important to pass on to friends and daughters that lumps come in all shapes and sizes.

What matters is that you've decided to live well now

Some women are so afraid of finding out that they have cancer that they deliberately delay diagnosis. Others stay quiet because they are terrified that they will lose their husband or partner along with a breast, or lose their chance of having children, or of forming a meaningful relationship if they are single.

If this was your choice, you may now be finding it hard to live with, especially if you believe your prognosis would be better if you had acted more swiftly.

Think of this. Some women choose to die rather than confront their fear. You are not one of them. However long it took, whatever your reasons for waiting, you found the courage to act. And you have now chosen to do the best you can to live well.

It doesn't matter how you came to this point. The best possible thing you can do is accept your choices and put them behind you.

YOU DON'T NEED A MEDICAL DEGREE TO SURVIVE

- There's a middle ground between playing the role of helpless bystander and carrying an unwelcome weight of medical responsibility
- When you have faith in the people who will be taking care of you there's no need to feel embarrassed about accepting their opinion
- Do as much or as little research as you need in order to feel comfortable

It used to be that all doctors were treated with absolute deference. No patient would have presumed to question his (it was rarely a 'her') diagnosis or treatment. If he told us we were simply being a hypochondriac, we believed him. If he told us we had a month to live, we believed that, too – and we may well have been obedient enough to live or die accordingly!

These days, few of us would be willing to play the role of helpless bystander in our own lives. However, there are some women who feel that the pendulum has swung too far in the opposite direction – that they are now expected to carry an unwelcome weight of medical responsibility.

Many books and websites dealing with breast cancer advocate gathering as much information as possible. Some women do exactly this and feel enormously reassured when they can understand and comment on every detail of their diagnosis and treatment. But this depth of knowledge isn't compulsory. For some people, too much information can be confusing and frightening, especially at a time when shock can make the instructions for making instant coffee seem like incomprehensible gibberish.

By coincidence, when I discovered my lump I was in the middle of writing a website which included a detailed and comprehensive section on breast cancer. At first I thought that being the best-informed non-medical patient in the universe would be a distinct advantage. Yet, in the end, I found that, at that time, details like tumour staging and oestrogen receptor status were of absolutely no help to me. My detailed knowledge did little but create occasional knots of unnecessary anxiety.

When you have faith in the people who will be taking care of you there's no need to feel embarrassed about accepting their opinion. For instance, my surgeon told me that one aspect of my treatment had been influenced by a recent study. When I mentioned this to a friend, she was astounded that I hadn't asked for details so that I could read it for myself. She would have wanted to; I most certainly didn't.

As far as I was concerned, my team understood the significance of the findings a lot better than I could ever hope to and were a lot better placed to decide whether the treatment would be appropriate for me. This was all I needed to know.

Beware the Internet

A little learning may be a dangerous thing, but throwing the Internet into the mix adds potential for total disaster.

There's certainly a lot of useful, practical and reassuring information out there, particularly at the world's official Cancer Council and leading breast cancer charity sites. Unfortunately, there's also a lot that you're better off without.

Shonky alternative sites are among the worst – especially those trying to persuade you to spend thousands of dollars on a miracle 'cure' by presenting page after page of 'genuine' medical disasters.

Don't go there! They can be of no benefit, but they can depress you for days.

WHAT WILL I LOOK LIKE?

- The mysterious mastectomy scar
- Many people assume we look a lot worse than we do
- When you have a choice of treatment, take your time to make the right decision for you

---

The position of my lump made it impossible to save my nipple, so there was never any question of a lumpectomy. It was then I realised that, despite having a head crammed with information, I had no idea what a mastectomy scar looked like.

I vaguely remembered catching a glimpse of my aunt's chest after a mastectomy some thirty years before – in my mind it looked as though her breast had been burned off with a blow torch. I must have been carrying round the idea that a breast was simply sliced off, leaving a big, round wound to scab over and scar.

When my doctor showed me a photograph of what the scar was really going to look like my relief was boundless. It looked like a picture of a child's chest – flat, but not even slightly repulsive.

Nothing to be ashamed of

Until someone discovers a treatment for breast cancer which doesn't involve surgical intervention, more than ten per cent of women in the western world will lose one or both breasts, or part of a breast. The fact that there are so many of us, yet so few people know what we look like, suggests that we are, at best, very shy and secretive or, at worst, embarrassed and ashamed.

I painted a 'topless topless' portrait of myself after I had had my breasts removed – and also allowed a friend to paint one in a very different style – because I think it's time post-mastectomy women came out of the closet.

Fear of gross disfigurement causes some women to delay seeking treatment. It fills husbands and partners with dread of what they're going to wake up with. And I'm sure that many people assume we look a lot worse than we do.

What's right for you

Until the 1970s, women undergoing surgery for breast cancer had no choice – they had what is known as a radical mastectomy. In this operation, the muscle of the chest wall and all of the lymph nodes under the arm are removed along with the breast.

A British surgeon eventually showed that the far less disfiguring modified radical mastectomy was just as effective for similar stages of disease. That meant the majority of women were able to retain the underlying muscle. This technique also spared more skin, which introduced the possibility of reconstruction.

In the past 15 years, surgery for early breast cancer has been scaled back even further with the introduction of lumpectomy or breast conservation surgery. While this is not always an option (as in my case), where it is possible it is just as effective as a mastectomy. If a competent surgeon offers a lumpectomy, choosing a mastectomy will not increase your chance of survival.

A reconstruction?

Breast reconstruction can make a huge difference to how you feel by helping you look good in your clothes without using a prostheses. However, it may involve one or more extra operations and, depending on the technique used, you may have a scar elsewhere on your body. Some women think it's worth it. Others don't.

If you're not sure, you don't have to rush into a decision. While some surgeons will perform reconstructive surgery at the time of the mastectomy, it can take place any time after healing. However, it's important to let your surgeon know if you might consider reconstruction at a later date as he or she may adjust the surgery slightly or consult a plastic surgeon as to the best place for the incision.

On a scale of 0 to 10, where 0 is not caring whether you have breasts or not and 10 is being unable to live without them, I reckon I score about a 4. I would hardly have had them removed by choice – but, when I realised that losing one was inevitable, my big fear was that my surgeon wouldn't remove both at the same time.

I knew with absolute certainty that I would never want reconstruction surgery. I'm too scared of both surgery and pain to have any sort of voluntary procedure. I had one ear pierced when I was 21 and I'm still trying to pluck up courage to get the other one done!

I have always found bras uncomfortable and chosen to go without one whenever propriety allowed, so the idea of a prosthesis was my ultimate nightmare. I knew in my heart that leaving hospital braless, wearing a T-shirt and feeling flat but symmetrical would give me the best possible chance of coping emotionally.

I met my surgeon for the first time having rehearsed a long and passionate speech to plead my cause. When I finally paused for breath, he showed me the mammogram of my 'healthy' breast. It was dotted with tiny points of calcification, any one of which might, apparently, have been malignant. It was not so bad that he would have recommended a double mastectomy unless I had raised the issue myself but, as I had, he felt that there was strong medical support for my request.

Surprising reactions

It's incredible how differently – and unpredictably – women react to breast surgery.

One friend, a dynamic and attractive woman in her early thirties, had a mastectomy a few months before I did and was always comfortable with the idea of wearing a prosthesis. Another, in her sixties, had a reconstruction at the time of her recent mastectomy. She was eager to put cancer behind her and felt that having only one breast would be too much of a reminder. A third friend, in her late thirties, left the option of a reconstruction open until several months after surgery. When she decided to go ahead, it was mainly because she spends a lot of time in a swimsuit and felt it would be easier.

Only you can possibly know your own priorities, how you feel about your body and what would work best for you.

Should you consider a double mastectomy?

When you're diagnosed with breast cancer you may feel you just couldn't face going through the whole experience again. You might want to get rid of both breasts at the same time; if one has betrayed you, why wouldn't the other one do the same?

Few surgeons would agree to a double mastectomy at this stage. A diagnosis of breast cancer is a hugely emotional experience and you can't necessarily trust your first reactions. After having time to think, and perhaps speaking to a counsellor about probable outcomes, most women decide to keep one breast after all.

5

SURGERY

- Emotional rather than physical pain
- Emotions out of control
- Life goes on
- Avoiding lymphoedema

One of the more surreal moments in my life was lying on an operating table, lifting the neck of my gown and saying goodbye to my breasts.

It was 6.30pm on Thursday, January 13th 2000. I was about to have a double mastectomy and lose all of the lymph nodes under my right arm.

I have to admit that, at that moment, my fear of pain overwhelmed any other consideration. My anaesthetist had been very reassuring about pain control, but her kind words served mainly to put pain at the top of my mind when I hadn't really thought about it before.

I've already admitted to being a total wimp, especially when it comes to anything to do with needles or cutting. I'm sure the real reason I chose natural childbirth for all four of my children was that I was less afraid of labour pains than having a needle in my spine for an epidural.

By the time I climbed on to the trolley I was imagining waking up to searing torments which no drug would be able to control. I had also convinced myself that the anaesthetic wouldn't work at all and that, apparently unconscious, I would be able to feel every flicker of the scalpel.

Naturally, I felt nothing. However, as soon as I regained consciousness, my enduring panic prompted me to described a twinge of discomfort as 'pain' to a nurse. To her credit, she took me at my word and promptly injected me with morphine. I knew as soon as it wore off that I hadn't really needed it. Oral painkillers were fine.

The real pain for most women, of course, is realising that part of you is gone forever.

Initially, I think that coming to terms with being breastless was a lot easier for me than for many. I had small breasts. I had had my children. I had no man in my life, which meant I only had one set of emotions to deal with. And I've always been happiest in jeans and a T-shirt.

The only clothes I had to discard were a few sports bras. If I'd gone home to drawers full of lacy lingerie and a wardrobe of low-cut dresses, or if I'd had yet to have children, I'm sure that the first glimpse of my washboard chest would have been infinitely more painful. As it was, I found the drainage tubes more disturbing than the actual wound. I just hated the thought of them. Even when the bulky dressing was removed to reveal rows of little white tabs marching across my chest I was more impressed by the neatness than appalled by the flatness.

It was to be several weeks before I experienced my first wave of profound sadness and loss. It only lasted a few minutes, but the strength of the emotion took me completely by surprise.

It went on happening from time to time, sometimes triggered by 'phantom nipple itch', when my hand would

You can move your arm!

While I was in hospital I became obsessed with recovering full movement in my right arm – the side from which lymph nodes had been removed. I couldn't stand the idea that cancer would continue to have power over me by limiting what I could do in the future.

From the day after the operation I started the regular shoulder-rolling and shrugging recommended in the guide provided by the hospital. It felt revolting – lots of hideous popping and squeaking – but, for once in my life, I persisted. I really believe it helped; there's now virtually no difference in the range of movement I have in each arm, even when I do yoga poses.

move automatically to where a nipple ought to be. There was the odd flash of total disbelief, as if I'd just woken from a dream and that my body was still just as it was. And I also found it sobering when, during radiotherapy, one of the technicians touched my chest gently as she got me into the right position. It felt quite sensuous – and then I realised with a shock that the mild sensation I was experiencing was as much as I could ever expect from what was once an erogenous zone.

Those feelings eventually passed. These days, the only time I'm really conscious of my chest is when I'm shopping for women's clothes. If that sounds odd, I've worn mostly boy's or men's clothes since I was a teenager – they fit my straight-up-and-down figure, long arms and broad shoulders better than female equivalents. Very occasionally, though, I need to find something a little more feminine and those empty, darted bosoms can be quite depressing. However, knowing that a local dressmaker can get rid of them in no time has made the experience much easier to handle.

Going home

I was well enough to leave on the third day after my surgery but decided to wait another 24 hours until the final drainage tube was removed.

I felt wonderfully well, almost frighteningly, optimistic. During a sleepless night I had written myself a new life plan. I could already move my arm enough to impress unsuspecting visitors. I had started planning my 'topless topless' painting and feeling that I might have a role to play in helping others to accept the way we look after our operations. In my T-shirt, I didn't even look noticeably different. The cancer, the operation – it all felt like no big deal.

The bruising on my chest and sides was, of course, spectacular, but the wounds were healing well. My surgeon made identical cuts on both sides of my chest, managing to remove all of the lymph nodes without any extra incisions. I was surprised by how well balanced I looked.

Then, when I got home, I discovered that the wound left by the last drainage tube was leaking and needed redressing. I made an appointment with the nurse at my local doctor's surgery and was kept waiting for half an hour because the receptionist had forgotten to tell her I was there.

My reaction shocked everyone, including me – it was as though someone had pulled a plug on my emotions.

"I had a double mastectomy three days ago and you can't even arrange a bloody appointment with a nurse," I screamed in a waiting room full of bemused and embarrassed people. I then rushed into the treatment room and collapsed in tears.

By the time I left, I was calm once again. However, this demonstration of emotions out of control was one of the issues that prompted me to see a counsellor. It was becoming increasingly obvious to me that I needed help with acknowledging and releasing my feelings rather than suppressing them until they erupted in an uncontrolled burst of anger, then quickly hammering a lid on them again.

Life goes on

I had booked a holiday for a week after the operation and was determined to go – I wanted a break before chemotherapy started. My eldest son had recently started learning to drive and was delighted with the opportunity to take the wheel for such a long distance, a trip of around five hours. I used one of my daughter's soft, duck-shaped pillows to protect myself from the pressure of the seat belt and felt OK, even if I looked a little old to be cuddling up to a stuffed toy.

I happened to be staying with a close friend who is also a doctor, which was especially reassuring, and my surgeon rang after a couple of days to see how I was going. The only problem I experienced was the amount of fluid collecting under my right arm – a normal occurrence after a mastectomy, but uncomfortable all the same.

I had had the fluid drained the day before I left but, by day three of the holiday, I felt as though I had a football under my right armpit. I actually needed to support the swelling as I walked around, so I decided to go to a local doctor to have it drained again.

He was wonderful. He insisted on giving me a local anaesthetic even though I didn't have a great deal of feeling in the area and it worked like a charm. While I couldn't say the first draining had been a painful experience, I was certainly aware of it and was not looking forward to having it done again. This doctor took his time and was extremely gentle. I felt nothing.

I had to have that side drained another four times – twice by my family doctor who, again, used a local anaesthetic, and twice by the nurse who had administered my chemotherapy. She didn't use anaesthetic but had a technique of injecting into the scar which, along with her amazing gentleness, meant, once again, I felt nothing at all.

Avoiding lymphoedema

Lymphoedema is the cause of the persistently swollen arm that some women experience after being treated for breast cancer.

You are at risk of developing lymphoedema if you have some or all of the lymph nodes removed from under your arm, or radiation to your armpit. It can develop at any time from immediately after surgery to 20 or more years later though it's most likely to strike in the first year. And, while estimates of the risk vary greatly, it is clear that the more treatment you've had, the greater the risk.

Lymph is a vital part of our defence system. Normally, it circulates throughout the body, draining from the arms and legs with the help of lymph nodes. When the lymph nodes are removed or damaged it is more difficult for the fluid to drain. As a result, lymphatic fluid can build up in the tissues.

Your surgeon will almost certainly remove some or all of the lymph nodes under your arm during surgery for breast cancer. In planning your treatment, your doctors need to know whether cancer cells have spread into the lymph nodes and, if so, how many nodes are affected. Unfortunately, the only way to find out is to examine them under a microscope, which means that some women find themselves in the frustrating position of suffering from lymphoedema as a result of having all of their perfectly healthy lymph nodes removed.

Sentinel node biopsy

A new technique called sentinel node biopsy, or sentinel node dissection, may offer an alternative. Here, the surgeon identifies the sentinel node – the first one likely to be affected if the cancer did spread – and removes this, perhaps with the two or three closest to it. If these prove to be free from cancer cells, other lymph nodes are unlikely to be affected and so are left in place. If they are not free, all of the other lymph nodes will be removed.

Trials so far have shown that the technique can reduce side-effects such as lymphoedema. It also seems to be as accurate when associated with relatively small breast cancers as more invasive testing. Of course, that doesn't mean it's 100 per cent accurate so, if you are considering sentinel node biopsy, you need to understand the risks as well as the benefits. You should also ensure that your surgeon is trained in this particular procedure.

Doing your best to avoid lymphoedema

Lymphoedema can be managed but there is no cure. There are, however, steps that you can take to prevent it. I have been fanatical!

If I did see any signs of lymphoedema – and, remember, it can happen years after surgery – I would seek out specialist advice immediately. Apparently, a special massage technique for lymphatic drainage can help considerably, but this is very different from every other type of therapeutic massage. The practitioner needs to learn from a physiotherapist with specific experience in this area.

The hospital where I had my radiotherapy runs a workshop on lymphoedema once a month for women who are at risk. Your doctor or hospital should be able to guide you to something similar if you have any concerns at all.

If you have symptoms, don't wait

The sooner you start to treat lymphoedema, the easier it is to manage. Signs to look out for are:

- a full sensation in the arm
- a feeling of tightness in the skin
- reduced flexibility in the hand or wrist
- a noticeable tightness in one sleeve
- noticing that a ring, bracelet or watch feels tighter

If you have any reason to believe that lymphoedema may be developing, see your doctor immediately and don't be fobbed off – specialist advice is vital.

Take good care of your arm

I never forget that lymphoedema can strike at any time so I continue to follow these recommendations to the letter.

- Act quickly to stop serious lymphoedema before it starts. Don't ignore even a slight increase in size or a constant ache in your arm or shoulder.

- Keep your arm spotlessly clean but don't use soap as it can dry the skin. Choose a soap-free cleanser – your pharmacist will be able to recommend one. Dry your arm gently but thoroughly, and be sure to include the skin between your fingers

- Avoid damaging the skin in any way. Knocks, cuts, sunburn, ordinary burns, sports injuries and insect bites are all potential sources of infection, and infection can cause lymphoedema. Try not to bite your nails and be careful with your cuticles. Never cut them – just ease them back with cotton wool on an orange stick. This also applies when you're having a professional manicure. Wear a thimble when you're sewing and gloves when you're gardening. If you're out in the countryside, wear a shirt with long sleeves.

- If you spot a rash or any redness or warmth which might indicate an infection see your doctor right away in case you need antibiotics. Treat any scratches, grazes, cuts or insect bites promptly to avoid infection by cleaning the area thoroughly and applying an antiseptic cream or lotion.

- Don't use your 'at risk' arm to carry heavy a heavy briefcase, suitcase, handbag or shoulder bag.

- Avoid vigorous, repetitive movements against resistance with the affected arm (a great reason never to scrub a floor again). At the very least, rest frequently.

- Where possible, don't allow anyone to measure your blood pressure, take blood or inject your 'at risk' arm. Don't assume that all medical professionals know about the risk of lymphoedema – you may need to explain. If both arms are at risk, it's usually possible to use a leg or foot. If there's no choice but to use your 'at risk' arm – in an emergency, for instance, or when you're having chemotherapy – don't panic. While it makes sense to reduce your chances of getting lymphoedema when you can, caution shouldn't get in the way of important treatment.

- Keep your arm as cool as possible in hot weather and stay out of saunas and hot tubs. Don't apply heating pads or hot compresses to your affected arm or to your neck, shoulder and back on the affected side.

- Avoid extreme temperature changes when bathing or washing dishes. Wear rubber gloves when you wash dishes or clothes.

- It is very important to keep your skin supple and moist. Moisturise at least once a day after your bath or shower.

- Protect your arm from sunburn by wearing long sleeves, staying in the shade where possible and wearing sunscreen when you can't.

- Eat a good, balanced diet with plenty of fibre and fluids but not too much salt or alcohol. You may hear that lymphoedema is high-protein oedema and wonder whether you should cut down on protein. Don't. Eating too little protein can actually increase the risk by weakening the connective tissue in your arm.

- Please don't smoke!

- Aim to stay within your healthiest weight range.

- If you're travelling by air, move around, exercise your arm gently when you can and drink plenty of water during the flight. If you already have swelling, wear a compression sleeve with a gauntlet or glove.

- Don't wear your clothes or jewellery too tight. You should take particular care with your bra – have it well fitted and avoid under-wiring if possible. Your skin should show no signs of redness or indentation when you take it off. If you have large breasts and wear a prosthesis, choose a lightweight one.

- Exercise, but do it moderately, starting slowly and increasing gradually. Your arm shouldn't ache with tiredness. If it does, it's a good idea to lie down and keep it elevated for a while. Gentle exercise like walking and swimming is important for lymph drainage. Never lift more than seven kilos.

- A properly-maintained electric razor is safer for removing hair from under your arm than safety razors, depilatories or abrasive mitts.

6

CHEMOTHERAPY

> - **There is a positive side**
> - **Take good care of yourself**
> - **Don't expect to feel sick**
> - **Losing your hair**

Chemotherapy has a terrible reputation. True, it can have side-effects that no-one would choose to endure, but it also has one 'side effect' that makes any suffering very worthwhile – a greatly increased chance of living a long and healthy life.

It's easy to lose touch with why you're having chemotherapy – to see it as some kind of punishment or torture that's being done to you rather than for you. Unfortunately, if you do, you could find yourself trapped in a vicious circle where negative feelings and depression compound the effects of your treatment.

There are a few strategies which might make the experience more bearable.

Something to look forward to

- *Do something you enjoy around the time of your treatment*
   Give yourself something to look forward to and you might just balance out that feeling of dread. For the first treatment, it's a good idea to plan your treat for the night before just in case you don't feel terrific afterwards. If

you find you feel fine and your treatment is in the morning, next time you could plan a great lunch or undemanding afternoon activity so that you still have the evening to rest.

- *Do something you enjoy while you're having the treatment*

  Your chemotherapy might well be administered through a drip – and sitting with a drip in your arm is a lot more bearable if you're doing something other than reading dog-eared hospital magazines. Start a gripping new novel the day before and you'll appreciate having a few hours to yourself to get on with it. Or, if you find it hard to concentrate on a book, at least take a couple of magazines you particularly enjoy.

- *If you work, forget about it*

  If you're flat out at work it's easy to resent every second of the time you're 'wasting' on your treatment. The amount of stress this will generate is enormous – especially if you end up spending more time at the hospital than you had allowed.

  It's easy to forget that your health is at stake, and nothing is more important. Tell yourself this fact over and over until you believe it, and until you're ready to treat your chemotherapy as a welcome step towards total recovery rather than an outrageous imposition.

- *Shut out the rest of the world*

  If you don't want to read, don't feel totally comfortable with the environment while you're having your treatment or you really don't want to talk to anyone, take an MP3 or CD player with you. It's a great way of keeping the world at bay. If music isn't distracting enough, try spoken-word recordings. CDs are available at many bookshops and most public libraries and a huge range of subjects is available including novels, non-fiction and recordings of comedy series. You might also find that a spiritual or motivational tape provides just the lift you need.

Another option is a portable DVD player – with headphones of course. TV series demand less concentration than films and, unlikely as it sounds, you might actually find yourself laughing at the comedies.

Take good care of yourself

Cancer cells are hard to kill because they're so similar to normal cells. One of their more distinctive characteristics is that they are actively growing and dividing; these are the kinds of cells targeted by chemotherapy.

Unfortunately, the friendly cells that make your hair grow, line your mouth and gut, carry oxygen around in your blood and protect you from infection are also growing and dividing. As yet, chemotherapy can't differentiate between the good and the bad.

As the cancer cells don't recover as quickly or as completely as the friendly cells they are less likely to survive the medication. But, as far as your body is concerned, there's a hell of a lot of rebuilding to be done during the course of your treatment. It makes sense to me that your body needs all the help it can get, along with top-quality materials for the job.

I had two courses of chemotherapy and, during both, I ate well, and supplemented my diet with good-quality and

While it's very important to drink plenty of fluids after your chemotherapy treatment, you may want to limit your drinks during any intravenous treatments – especially the longer ones.

Going to the loo is a complicated procedure, and some nurses prefer that you don't move around while the drip is in place.

My Taxol treatment took around six hours to administer, with three hours on the drug itself. It also began with a litre of saline solution. The first time, I cheerfully sipped away on endless cups of herbal tea delighted to be putting so much fluid into my system. This was not a good idea – especially as I was sitting next to a burbling, aerated fish tank!

very comprehensive vitamin, mineral and antioxidant supplements. I also took vitamin E, and three to six grams of vitamin C with bioflavonoid. This I had as powder dissolved in fruit juice.

Whether or not to take vitamins is a controversial topic. The reality is that nutrition is still a very young science and there simply hasn't been enough research to provide many definite answers. We're told to discuss our choices with our doctors, which would make sense if we could be sure that our doctors would be sympathetic, or at least open minded.

Unfortunately, many continue dismiss any treatment which could be even loosely described as 'complementary'. Others may be reluctant to voice a different view because they don't have research to back up their advice and, sad to say, they also have a justifiable fear of being sued.

Since I had my treatment, some scientists have suggested that antioxidants such as vitamins C, A, D and E might interfere with the effect of radiation treatment. Now, I might cut them while I was actually undergoing radiotherapy, though probably not at any other time.

I've long been a fan of vitamin C and for years I've taken huge amounts to fend off the effects of a cold. It seems to work for me (obviously – I'd hardly keep doing it if it didn't!) Evidence for this effect seems to be mixed, though supporters argue that the doses tested in the little research that has been carried out are generally far too low. Yes, it can cause diarrhoea and stomach cramps when taken in quantity though, in my experience, the body adapts easily if you increase the dose gradually. It has also been said that most of a large dose will be excreted, unchanged, in the urine.

Nevertheless, there is some evidence that vitamin C helps to protect against colds and infection.

Chemotherapy leaves you particularly vulnerable to infection because it lowers your white blood count. Your body is also less able to fight back, so that even a relatively minor infection could result in hospitalisation for intravenous antibiotics. Given these circumstances, anything that helps resist infection sounds good to me. During my treatment, I didn't get a single cold or bout of flu and I stayed well even when my whole family was sneezing and coughing all around me. Did vitamin C help? Who can say? But I still take a gram every day.

Doesn't chemotherapy make you sick?

The first symptom of chemotherapy you're likely to think of is nausea. However, thanks to modern anti-nausea medication, most women will cruise through with very little discomfort. As I had had four children without more than a passing nod to morning sickness I fully expected to be one of them.

Unfortunately, it wasn't to be. For some reason, my first course of chemotherapy made me very sick indeed, even when I was on the highest possible dose and combination of anti-emetic drugs. I think I may actually be allergic to the anti-emetics. Whatever the reason, when I had to be admitted to hospital for intravenous fluids after my third treatment, my oncologist decided not to go ahead with the fourth.

The treatment I was having, cyclophosphamide doxorubicin, or 'AC' as it is know, has a reputation for being one of the least pleasant but, even so, I was told it was very unusual to react so violently. I must admit that I felt a bit sceptical – after all, wasn't this what chemotherapy was about? But, since then I've spoken to many other women who had had the same treatment without anything more dramatic than mild and temporary discomfort.

The message is not to expect nausea – it probably won't happen. If it does, there are usually ways to make it as manageable and short-lived as possible.

- Try your hardest to keep up your fluid intake. It took me a while to find a drink I could tolerate and that turned out to be weak fruit tea with a slice of ginger. Ginger does have an anti-emetic effect, so ginger tea is a good place to start. You could also try a lemon and honey drink or water with a squeeze of lemon or grapefruit juice. For some reason, plain water can be quite undrinkable. To me, all water tasted as if someone had added artificial sweetener – revolting!

- Have all of your drinks at room temperature and take tiny sips.

- Homemade soup is a great way of eating and drinking simultaneously. Potato soup (recipe on page 146) is about as bland as you can get, and it kept me going for a couple of days after my first treatment.

- Stewed apple or pear cooked with a little extra water to make it really juicy is another good and non-threatening combination of food and drink.

- When you feel hungry, eat small amounts of plain food only. After four days of eating nothing at all, I was so excited by a hunger pang that I continued eating after my stomach said 'stop'. I was back to square one in an instant, unable to eat again for the rest of the day.

- Don't get too hungry. Hunger can be quite nauseating in itself – keep a packet of plain crackers handy when you're out of the house.

Taxol

My second chemotherapy cycle, Taxol, was very different in its effect from AC. It generally doesn't cause nausea but, given my history, I was given medication anyway. I took it once then decided to try without it and was fine, not nauseous at all. I did get some aches and pains – in my legs, mainly – but they weren't bad enough to interfere with normal life. I even spent a weekend in the country with my daughter just two days after one treatment. I'd forgotten about it when I made the booking but decided to go ahead and was glad I did. I even managed an hour-long walk, though my knees were shaking a bit on the steeper sections of the climb!

Another Taxol side effect is numbness in the fingertips and toes. I was warned that I might have difficulty fastening buttons by the end of my treatment but the worst I experienced was a slight and occasional tingling.

Staying well

When you start chemotherapy you will probably be presented with a list of possible side effects. It can make frightening reading unless you remember that these really are *possible*, not inevitable.

Apart from the short term nausea associated with AC, I experienced very little discomfort. I didn't feel much more tired than usual, my energy levels stayed high and, apart from some spicy dishes making my tongue feel sore, I didn't have any mouth problems. I also stayed exactly the same weight throughout my treatment. Not everyone is quite so lucky but there's really no need to expect the worst.

Losing your hair

For many of us, losing our hair is the most traumatic side effect of chemotherapy.

I wasn't sure how I would react, or whether I would want wear a wig. I thought I wouldn't – then, when my hair started falling out in massive clumps, I panicked and decided I had to have a wig after all.

As I watched myself in the mirror trying on impossibly inappropriate styles, then taking the wigs off to find half of my hair still inside them and the rest lying thin and flat on my head, I experienced one of the lowest moments in the whole process of having cancer.

I couldn't believe it was really happening – that I really was going to be bald. I have always had full, messy hair to balance my 'strong' features. Suddenly I felt totally exposed and vulnerable. I had a wave of feeling that I simply couldn't cope – an overwhelming helplessness that I'd managed to avoid even when I had my surgery.

Eventually, we found a wig that even I had to admit looked very realistic and was reasonably close to my old style. It was something I could wear and without feeling ridiculous, so I had my safety net.

That night, the children had a wonderful time shaving my head. As soon as they had finished I felt strangely liberated – I discovered that I could cope better with being bald than with balding. I was also starting to think that the wig may not be such a great idea for me.

I was right. I never wore the wig or even a hat apart from a beanie when I was cold. Facing the world with a bald head made me feel courageous and strong, a reminder that I could stare down my worst demons. That's what made it right for me.

I know this isn't typical – I must be more of an exhibitionist than I realised! Most women are more comfortable staying covered, whether with a scarf, turban or wig. And, these days, wigs are generally undetectable –

One of the most memorable experiences of my treatment was going to see 'Wit', a play about a woman with cancer.

For most of the performance, she wore nothing but a hospital gown and a baseball cap. Then, in one of the play's more dramatic moments, she removed the cap to reveal her own shaved head as she spoke about the humiliation of losing all one's hair.

The fact that my own bald skull was glowing softly – and very obviously – in the semi-darkness just a couple of metres away must have made those lines particularly difficult to deliver!

you'll even have trouble spotting them in the oncology unit where you know most of the women have no hair.

I don't think the 'naturalness' of a wig has anything to do with cost. The one I bought was very inexpensive – thank goodness the woman who sold it to me persuaded me away from the phenomenally-priced human hair wigs which I thought I would simply have to have. She told me that the latest synthetic wigs are just as realistic (a claim backed up by the few people I have ever put my wig on for) but very much lighter and easy to wear. They're also much easier to care for.

The wigs you can spot tend to be those which are the wrong colour.

You may be told to buy your wig before your hair falls out so that you can match your natural shade. This is not always a good idea, especially if your own hair is dark. As treatment progresses, your eyebrows and eyelashes will probably fade, thin out or even disappear altogether, giving your face the effect of being much paler than usual. This could then make your own hair colour look unnaturally dark. Go for a lighter, softer shade and you'll be more likely to keep your chemotherapy to yourself.

7

RADIOTHERAPY

> - **Tedious but not traumatic**
> - **Be careful what you put on your skin**
> - **Don't expect to suffer – you probably won't**

For me, the worst thing about radiotherapy was the inconvenience. By the time I'd driven to the hospital, had the treatment and driven home again I'd lost over two hours out of each working day – not the best way to run a business.

However, I realise that's nothing compared with the inconvenience some women have to suffer. As radiotherapy is available only in major hospitals, anyone living outside a city has either a huge amount of travelling to cope with or needs to spend weekdays living away from the family. The pressure must be immense.

I found the treatment itself to be tedious but not traumatic. Each time the machine was switched on I either let my mind drift in a vague meditation for a minute or focused on how it was helping me to heal. As with chemotherapy, it's easy to see radiotherapy as a form of punishment but you're sure to feel better if you can regard it as a helpful friend.

In all I had 25 treatments. This went over the Easter holiday and, as the unit closed every second Friday for the machine to be serviced, it took just about six weeks. Everything went brilliantly, with only a faint reddening of

> While you're having your radiotherapy treatment, remember to wear a top and skirt or trousers rather than a dress. This way you will save yourself from the embarrassment of trying to keep a back-fastening hospital gown closed over your knickers.
>
> As you will need to apply moisturising cream regularly, you will probably want to stick to separates at the weekend and on your days off too. It makes taking care of your skin that much easier.

my skin until week five. Then I suddenly developed nasty, linear blisters under my arm.

The radiologist spotted them first – as I haven't had any sensation under my arm since surgery I hadn't even noticed they were there.

The rule at my hospital was to put nothing on the skin apart from sorbolene. I understand that this is because anything containing metals can increase the damage done by the radiation.

I have sworn by lavender oil for burns since I scalded my arm badly and found that it had a close to miraculous effect on my skin; I don't even have a scar. I felt confident that a pure essential oil would be OK and, as I didn't want to be told no, I took fate into my hands and slapped on undiluted lavender oil on four times a day.

By the following day the blisters had taken a dramatic turn for the better – healing without bursting. The radiologists were amazed, but I still didn't own up to what I had done. I felt too 'naughty'.

For me, lavender oil was like a miracle cure, though it may not work for everyone. The problem with radiotherapy seems to be that, if something doesn't suit your skin, it can actually make the effects much worse. That's why I hesitate to recommend lavender oil unconditionally. You may want to discuss it with your radiologist or try it on a tiny area – perhaps right at the beginning of your treatment before any blistering starts.

Naturally, I was focused on the end of the treatment and, once the 25th session was over, heaved a huge sigh of relief. However, when I saw the nurse for a final check, she told me that the radiation can go on working in the skin for up to two weeks after treatment stops and that I could expect the reddening to deepen.

I was bitterly disappointed; in fact, this was one of the few times during my treatment that I felt depressed. I had thought the worst was over. In fact, the worst was to come.

The skin continued to redden as I had been warned, and I also started to get eruptions that seemed immune to lavender oil. I had a fever for a couple of days, and what I thought were mosquito bites on the top of my leg even though it was in the middle of winter and I was a bit mystified as to how a mosquito could get through so many layers of clothing! My chest felt hot to the touch and was covered in infected blisters, so it was both ferociously itchy and incredibly sore at the same time.

It sounds so obvious now, but it was only when the 'mosquito bites' spread over much of the right side of my body and further down my legs that it dawned on me that this might not just be a reaction to the radiotherapy.

In fact, I had a generalised skin infection which antibiotics put right in a couple of days. As an aside, as antibiotics can destroy the 'good' bacteria in your gut along with the 'bad', I also took acidophilus tablets to help replace them. The most obvious benefit of taking acidophilus is not getting thrush.

Redness, itching and blistering could all be symptoms of radiotherapy, and I had no idea about the degree of discomfort I should expect. If I had seen my doctor sooner, I would probably have escaped with very minor problems. Once again, I'd say don't expect to suffer. See a doctor or your specialist as soon as you feel more than a little discomfort and you will probably find that something simple can be done to relieve it.

8

THE CANCER CLUB

- United by fear
- Taking sensible precautions
- Don't take the news at face value

Once you've heard a doctor say 'yes' to one of the most scary words in the language you've become a member of the Cancer Club.

The most powerful force uniting its members is fear.

In the first few moments, there's the fear that you've just been given a death sentence. Then there's the fear of treatment and its side effects. Fear of pain. Fear of what effect cancer is going to have on your relationships and your family. And, when all of your treatment is over, fear that the cancer will come back.

However far along the track members may be, we will always be on the lookout for a magical formula or process that will guarantee we stay cancer free – a new drug, a new form of conventional treatment or a more alternative approach. It's important to remember that the vast majority of women who are diagnosed with breast cancer will not have a recurrence, including women who make no attempt at all to improve an unhealthy lifestyle. But I also believe that there are steps we can take to give ourselves the best possible chance of staying well.

Practicalities

It's unlikely that there is one single cause of breast cancer but various factors have been investigated as a possibility. Results vary according to which research paper you're reading, but there do seem to be some sensible precautions we can take.

- Don't smoke, and avoid smoky areas.

- Eat a wide range of wholesome foods.

- Avoid additives, preservatives and processed foods. Research suggests that some of the worst offenders are ham, salami and other preserved meats.

- Drink alcohol only in moderation (there's more about this on page 75).

- Take some form of regular exercise.

- Maintain a healthy weight.

Don't take the news at face value

When you've been there, it's only natural that any mention of cancer in the news will jump out like a flashing neon sign to grab your attention. The problem is that, while most media reports are not untruthful, they can present a picture which is misleading enough to cause unnecessary fear and confusion.

I've included the example below in case you're interested in how this can happen, and also because I remember how relieved I was when, by chance, I learned more about how research is reported. When you're feeling raw and vulnerable it's easy to get tied up in the detail of trying to do the right thing. This information helped me to stop panicking quite so readily and keep things a bit more in perspective – at least in the short term.

If you're not interested in the detail, just skip to the next chapter – but please be aware that you could save yourself a lot of heartache by checking with your doctor before you take any news report about cancer too seriously. If you do read on, let me make it very clear that I only used breath mints to make a point – I have never seen or heard of any link between breath mints and cancer in any way, shape or form!

So, imagine seeing a headline that says:

Breath mints increase risk of breast cancer by 13 per cent!

If you were someone who sucked a lot of breath mints you would have every right to be worried. But there's a lot the headline isn't saying and, when you're aware of that, you're a lot less likely to panic.

What kind of risk are they talking about?

You've probably heard that, if a woman lives to the age of 85, her risk of getting breast cancer is one in nine, or 11 per cent. This is **absolute** risk. Glancing at the headline, it would be easy to think that the 13 per cent increase would take that risk from 11 per cent to 24 per cent.

In fact, the increase is much more likely to be in terms of **relative** risk – in other words, that women sucking breath mints were 13 per cent more likely to get breast cancer than those who weren't. In this case, we're looking at 13 per cent **of** 11 per cent rather than **plus** 11 per cent, which is a percentage rise of just 1.43. It's still an increase, but a jump from 11 to 12.43 per cent is very different from 11 to 24 per cent.

Even a tiny increase would probably be enough to persuade us to bin the breath mints, but what if those statistics were associated with medication of some kind? When a link between hormone replacement therapy and breast cancer broke in the media, many women stopped taking their HRT medication immediately, precisely because the risk sounded so much higher than it actually is. Of course, they may have decided to forego the medication anyway but, had the risk been explained more clearly and reported in a less sensationalist way, they would have been spared much of the fear. They could also have made their decision in a much more calm and rational frame of mind.

'Absolute' versus 'relative' risk can also raise false hopes by making medication sound more effective than it is. Once again, it's important to understand a media report's terms of reference. If your doctor doesn't rush to prescribe a new drug that sounded fantastic in the newspaper, there could be a very good reason. Don't be afraid to ask.

What were they studying?

Were the studies done using people or animals? Researchers are eager to share their findings the moment they sound promising – sometimes before they have been thoroughly tested on humans.

How big was the study?

Asking 20,000 women who have breast cancer whether they suck breath mints will give a more meaningful result than asking 20. It sounds so obvious it's easy to assume that a report is based on a good-sized sample. It may not be.

Did the people being studied tell the truth?

We can't monitor people 24 hours a day. Researchers often have to base their conclusions on what their subjects tell them, and this can lead to all kinds of problems.

If the study is retrospective, memory is likely to be a factor. People might have no idea of how long they've been sucking breath mints or how many a day they were sucking, say, a year ago but feel they must say something because they've agreed to be part of the research.

Because we're human, reporting can also be affected by what we think people want to hear, or by the picture we like to present of ourselves. If we think that sucking breath mints suggests we're careful about oral hygiene we might, perhaps even subconsciously, push the number up a bit. On the other hand, if researchers were asking about smoking, we might feel self-conscious about how many cigarettes we actually smoke and push the number down.

Have the researchers taken other factors into account?

If the women who developed breast cancer after sucking breath mints had been using them to mask the smell of cigarette smoke you could probably take the mints out of the equation.

Have there been any previous studies?

If a number of different studies are all suggesting a link between breath mints and breast cancer there is more likely to be some kind of risk than if one study is swimming against the tide.

Is the report from a trustworthy source?

Generally, the stories that catch our eye in the media are taken from papers published in scientific journals. These papers have been 'peer reviewed' – evaluated by other experts in field – before they are published, so they're more likely to be credible than those which haven't. It helps to know which you're reading.

Who funded the research?

Without delving too deeply into the murky depths of conspiracy theories, it's a fact that most research is funded by someone these days, even research carried out in apparently impartial places like universities.

Research is expensive and the money has to come from somewhere; as long as the interest is clearly stated and the results are accurately reported, this isn't necessarily a problem. But it doesn't hurt to be aware of a connection.

For instance, I wonder how many people realise that research into the effectiveness of the hugely successful and surprisingly meat-heavy CSIRO Total Wellbeing Diet was funded by Dairy Australia and Meat and Livestock Australia? This fact in itself doesn't mean that the research was in any way skewed or inaccurate, but I think most of us would like to know about it.

9

FOOD

- Indulge yourself with the best of everything
- Easing into eating well
- Should you become a vegetarian?
- Should you drink juice?
- Quick, easy, healthy food
- How much water?

You might read this chapter and think I have a very peculiar attitude to food. If you do, that's fantastic. You are one of the women who see food as food rather than some sort of emotional explosive device. If you decide to change your diet, you will do it for rational reasons and you will do it with ease.

On the other hand, you may understand exactly what I'm talking about. If so, I really hope I can inspire you with my own experience.

Taking control

Diet is often the first thing people look to change when they're diagnosed with a life-threatening disease. Perhaps that's because diet feels like the one thing we can actually control. Unfortunately for most women, the idea that it's easy to control what we eat is a myth – any diet can be fraught with danger.

Many of us have an extraordinarily complex relationship with food well before breast cancer enters our lives. Most of us would like to weigh less – and, hard as non-Cancer Club members find it to believe, having cancer doesn't change this fact. Most of us have tried to follow diets or cut down on how much we eat in order to lose weight. Many of have experienced failure, consoling ourselves with chocolate, chips or pizza and feeling depressed, inadequate and guilty.

Imagine, then, the potential for guilt, misery and despair if you don't stick to a diet which you believe could be helping to save your life.

My own relationship with food has been more extreme than most. I suffered from various combinations of anorexia and bulimia for 14 years until pregnancy forced me to take better care of myself for my child's sake.

Before cancer, I still binged occasionally – once a month, maybe. Sometimes I'd make myself vomit, sometimes I didn't. Either way, I hated myself afterwards. I felt weak, worthless and out of control.

So many 'you can cure cancer'-type books treat food as though it is purely a means of staying alive. As if, once we have a life-threatening disease, our drive to survive will totally override our cravings, our love of certain foods and the emotions bound up in food and eating – and as if we will suddenly have no problem with following a rigid eating plan.

I find it hard to imagine any greater pressure. If you have ever eaten chocolate because you're fearful, anxious, bored, lonely, angry or depressed it's not very likely that sipping celery juice is going to satisfy your craving for comfort food when you're experiencing the turmoil of cancer. But the fact that you can't be perfect doesn't mean you should feel totally defeated. There are very good reasons for improving your diet where you can, but that doesn't mean you have to make your life a misery.

Move up the scale of health

It is well documented that the quality and types of foods you eat influence your general health. For instance, we're all familiar with the well-established links between eating large amounts of saturated fats and the incidence of heart disease. So, if a good diet can help you stay well, it seems reasonable to assume that good food can also help your body to heal.

When you're recovering from surgery or undergoing chemotherapy or radiotherapy, your body needs all the help it can get. Damage to healthy tissue is inevitable, and the nutrients you provide as food will support your body in the rebuilding process.

When your treatment is over, you want to give yourself the best possible chance of living a long and healthy life. That makes it even more important for you to find a way of eating healthily that you genuinely enjoy.

That doesn't mean being extreme.

Using a 1-10 scale again, if 1 is someone who lives on fast food take-aways and chocolate biscuits and 10 is someone who follows the most stringent, natural, healthy eating plan, you can feel pretty good about yourself if you move from a 2 to a 6. Or a 4 to an 8. Or even a 1 to a 2!

So where do you start? I think the most important place to begin is where most of us come unstuck – the foods we like best.

Indulge yourself

Have you ever read the word 'diet' and instinctively reached for chocolate to calm your nerves? Asked to see the dessert menu before you order your main course? Or eaten a whole packet of biscuits 'because they were there'? If you have, you'll understand why I think it's a good idea to sort out the cravings first. Until I'm absolutely assured that I'm not condemning myself to a life of misery and deprivation, I can't begin to think about serious eating.

We all have our own obsessions. I could spend a day sitting next to a plate of pizza or steaming hot chips without touching them, but I can't have chocolate in the house. A friend of mine would trample the finest Belgian truffles into the ground to get to cheese and olives. We're all different. And sometimes our obsession changes from day to day.

My belief is this – whatever it is you feel you can't live without, you don't have to try.

Treats you can enjoy every day

If you love coffee, you'll be delighted to hear that, after studying 85,987 women over a period of 22 years, scientists in America concluded that drinking coffee does not increase the risk of breast cancer.

That said, there's no escaping the fact that caffeine is a mild stimulant; too much can raise your blood pressure slightly, increase your heart rate and give you the 'jitters'.

So what's too much? It's hard to be precise when 'cup of coffee' covers everything from a weak latte to a triple strength espresso, but the general consensus seems to be that two or even three cups a day should be OK.

In the same study, tea also gets the all-clear, again when drunk 'in moderation'. And, in caffeine terms at least, there was no evidence of a link between breast cancer and chocolate. Hooray.

I used to think of red wine as another positive treat, and there is continuing support for theory that drinking moderate quantities of red wine can protect against heart disease. However, recent studies which appear to link alcohol consumption with an increased risk of breast and other types of cancer have prompted many organisations to amend their recommendations to either no alcohol at all or, for women, no more than one standard drink a day.

That doesn't necessarily mean one glass. A standard measure is just 100ml – just four tablespoons! Pour that into one of the fishbowl-size wine glasses that are so popular these days and it will barely touch the sides. If you do decide to treat yourself occasionally, relax and enjoy it…just be sure you've chosen the right-sized glass.

Enjoy yourself when you go out

As long as you don't go out every day, you can afford a little indulgence when you socialise. Choose your favourite foods and enjoy them to the full. If you can eat moderately, wonderful. If you go overboard, so what?

Life is about joy, fun and happiness – and that means having things to look forward to. Special occasions all seem to revolve around food and you need to be able to enjoy them wholeheartedly. Have the best possible time and get back to healthier eating as soon as you can.

At home, I eat mostly vegan food because I happen to love it and feel better when I'm not eating a lot of animal products.

Some of my friends enjoy creating vegan meals, or eating in vegan restaurants. Others just treat me as a non meat eater and prepare food with some egg or dairy products, or choose mainstream restaurants. At their homes I eat the vegetarian food they have provided. At the restaurant, I choose a dish without meat. I have dessert, and generally a glass of wine. I don't feel 'different' or alienated, or that I'm banned from enjoying myself. I want to stay well, but not at the expense of all the joy in my life.

After cancer I started to follow the 'enjoy the best to the full' strategy I talk about below and I was amazed to discover how well it works. For the first time in as long as I can remember I've actually enjoyed chocolate – a food I've always claimed to love, but have rarely tasted because I was always feeling guilty, worrying about whether I was going to eat 'too much' or, if I had already eaten my idea of too much, what I was going to eat next.

Nothing but the best

Just about every food you crave has a couple of healthier approximations which might hit the spot. If they don't, indulge in whatever it is you want so badly, but make sure it's the very best of its kind.

Buying the best can work for us on a number of different levels.

- If it's more expensive, you will be less tempted to 'buy up big'.
- Superior ingredients, flavour and texture should make it more satisfying than cheaper substitutes.
- It's easier to turn your treat into an occasion.

If you are a 'binger', you need to be in the right frame of mind before you indulge. This treat has nothing to with what you deserve or what you don't deserve. You are not eating because you are angry, disappointed, depressed or anxious, even though any of these emotions may have triggered the craving. Once you have made the decision to eat the food you're hanging out for, it's time to focus on the pleasure it will bring.

That means starting with a few basics.

Buy only as much as you can eat without feeling guilty

Satisfying your craving is about making yourself feel better, not worse. If your craving is for something that only comes in a bigger packet than you want to eat, make sure you can share it out before you start eating. If you have no-one to share it with, break off or set aside the right quantity for you and throw the rest in a litter bin on your way home.

This is not a waste of money. This is your favourite food – of course you're going to find it impossible to resist! Worse still, when I've bought large sizes and promised myself I'd eat a bit and save the rest till later, instead of enjoying the amount I feel comfortable with eating, I spend the whole time worrying about whether I'm going to give in and eat more. And, of course I always do. Then I feel guilty, angry with myself and out of control. This is the real waste of money.

Don't eat your treat on the way back from the shop

If necessary, lock it in the boot so that you won't be tempted.

When you get home, don't start eating until you can enjoy your treat completely. Don't read, watch TV or have half an eye on the children. Relish every mouthful, tasting every exquisite flavour. Remind yourself of why you're eating – for pleasure. The irony of bulimia and, I suspect, other forms of binge eating, is that you don't actually enjoy what you're eating at all because it's too loaded with emotion and worry.

When you've finished, do something that signals the end of the experience, such as cleaning your teeth.

Take the time to enjoy feeling satisfied, and to feel really pleased with yourself. You have proved to yourself that you can treat yourself to your favourite food and enjoy it in a controlled and reasonable way.

What's your weakness?

Sometimes a healthier alternative is enough, sometimes it just has to be the real thing. Either way, enjoy.

Chocolate, biscuits or cake

- Try a healthy treat like the fruit crumble on page 154
- Spread chocolate hazelnut spread on a slice of good quality bread
- Buy a small quantity of superb chocolate or your favourite biscuits or cake, relish every mouthful – and don't feel guilty.

Ice cream
- Eat a fat-free, all-natural fruit bar.
- Make a fruit smoothie – see page 155.
- Choose a single serve of good quality sorbet or gelato.
- Find the richest, most creamy and extravagant version of your favourite flavour, relish every mouthful - and don't feel guilty.

Hot chips
- Make your own by cutting up potatoes (skin on) then spreading them on a baking sheet. Drizzle on a little olive oil, sprinkle with sea salt then bake in a hot oven until they're crisp and brown. Or try the spicy potatoes on page 152.
- Oven-bake frozen chips.
- Buy a small serve of chips from your favourite take-away, relish every mouthful - and don't feel guilty.

Savoury snacks
- Unsalted nuts are great – pistachios in their shells have some salt, but they take so long to eat you're unlikely to go overboard!
- Make your own chips by thinly slicing potatoes, sweet potatoes, parsnips or other root vegetables and tossing them in a little olive oil. Spread them over a baking sheet, sprinkle with sea salt and spices such as chilli if you like, then bake them until they're crisp.
- Nibble on baked pretzels – they're salty enough to give the impression of chips.
- Buy a small packet of whatever it is that you can't live another minute without, relish every mouthful – and don't feel guilty

Pizza

- Make your own from the recipe on pages 149
- When only a takeaway will do, order your favourite flavour and share it. Have a slice yourself, relish every mouthful – and don't feel guilty

Cheese

There are some who suggest eating low-fat cheeses like cottage cheese and ricotta. If you love 'real' cheese, this is like trying to stem a craving for chocolate mud cake with a dry cracker. They just aren't the same animal.

I suggest you stay with your favourite cheeses but limit the amount you eat, both in quantity and frequency.

- If you have been in the habit of sprinkling grated cheddar around freely, you could find that a little Parmesan provides a good flavour with far less fat.

- If you eat cheese by the block, cut down the size of each serving and make sure that you're really enjoying the cheese, not letting it get lost in other flavours. Ready-sliced real cheese (as opposed to processed slices) is great for portion control – I know I couldn't slice cheese that thinly yet it's usually as much as you'd need in a sandwich.

- When you're cooking lasagne, moussaka or other cheesy dishes, you could try using ricotta or cottage cheese to add bulk and then sprinkling on Parmesan, pecorino or another strongly-flavoured hard cheese for extra flavour.

- Use Parmesan or other strongly-flavoured cheeses for sauces and you'll need to use much less.

Easing into eating well

Are there benefits associated with eating organically-grown food? I look at it this way.

Apple One was grown in a pest-free orchard and picked just a few days ago. It's fresh, tasty and has no trace of chemicals.

Apple Two has been sprayed with chemicals repeatedly since it was a bud. It was picked, coated in wax to make it look more shiny and held in cold storage for over a year before reaching the greengrocer where you bought it.

It's hard to believe that Apple One isn't better for you, and now there seems to be some evidence to support it. Research led by the University of Newcastle and involving scientists in Britain, France and Poland showed that organic carrots, apples, peaches and potatoes have greater concentrations of vitamin C and other nutrients.

Organic farming is also better for the environment, of course, so the only argument against organic food that I can see is the cost. Compared item-by-item with non-organic produce, the difference is enough to reduce any woman without a private income to tears. However, I'm not convinced the gap is so dramatic when you compare actual value. I shop for organic fruit and vegetables every week and I find I that I rarely throw anything away. Things seem to stay fresh for longer – perhaps because they haven't already spent months in storage. And anything appropriate that's starting to look even a bit tired goes into the juicer.

However, if you can't afford or don't want to pay for an all-organic diet, you can still reduce your chemical load by shopping strategically.

The not-for-profit Environmental Working Group, an American research and advocacy organisation, tested dozens of conventionally-grown fruits and vegetables for pesticide residues. As you can see from the list below, they found that some absorb far less than others. So, if you're on a budget, it would make sense to buy, say, ordinary onions and broccoli but organic strawberries and lettuce.

I also choose organic grains – rice, rolled oats, barley – and buy organic bread wherever possible.

RANK	FRUIT OR VEGETABLE	SCORE
1 (worst)	Peaches	100 (highest pesticide load)
2	Apples	96
3	Capsicums	86
4	Celery	85
5	Nectarines	84
6	Strawberries	83
7	Cherries	75
8	Lettuce	69
9	Grapes – imported	68
10	Pears	65
11	Spinach	60
12	Potatoes	58
13	Carrots	57
14	Green Beans	55
15	Chillis	53
16	Cucumbers	52
17	Raspberries	47
18	Plums	46

19	Oranges	46
20	Grapes – domestic	46
21	Cauliflower	39
22	Tangerine	38
23	Mushrooms	37
24	Cantaloupe	34
25	Lemon	31
26	Honeydew melon	31
27	Grapefruit	31
28	Winter squash	31
29	Tomatoes	30
30	Sweet potatoes	30
31	Watermelon	25
32	Blueberries	24
33	Papaya	21
34	Eggplant	19
35	Broccoli	18
36	Cabbage	17
37	Bananas	16
38	Kiwi fruit	14
39	Asparagus	11
40	Peas – frozen	11
41	Mangoes	9
42	Pineapples	7
43	Sweet corn – frozen	2
44	Avocado	1
45 (best)	Onions	1 (lowest pesticide load)

Reproduced from the Environmental Working Group website www.ewg.org

Vegetarian?

From a health point of view, arguments about vegetarianism have raged for years. While some studies indicate that vegetarians are generally healthier and live longer, others suggest that no meat means too little protein and iron.

And, of course, being vegetarian doesn't automatically mean you eat well. There's no meat in chocolate, ice cream, four-cheese pizza or chips!

I've been vegetarian or vegan for most of my adult life but it has made very little difference to the quality of the food I ate; I was vegetarian most of the time I was bulimic.

My decision not to eat meat or, where reasonably possible, any animal products, is less about health than animal cruelty, particularly the cruelty associated with intensive farming.

These days, if I did eat meat, I would choose organic wherever possible and avoid processed meats like salami and bacon, as well as any which have been charred in the cooking. Preservatives and the compounds formed when meat is cooked at high temperatures have both been put forward as possible carcinogens.

The benefits of juice

Juice features heavily in many healing diets. In some it seems to be credited with something close to magical powers. It's certainly a wonderful way of ingesting vitamins and minerals – especially if you're finding it difficult to eat solid food, or if you simply don't like raw

If you do decide to go the juice route, I would say the first thing to look for in a juicer is ease of cleaning. I borrowed an older model from a friend and used it once only. The cleaning process was so laborious and time-consuming that I just couldn't face using it again. By contrast, the one I bought – a Breville Juice Fountain Professional – is brilliant. As long as you do it immediately, running water is all it takes to clean parts other than the filter and that just needs a quick brush. The whole process takes no more than a couple of minutes.

vegetables. However, nothing is compulsory. Many women have lived for years after breast cancer without doing more than mixing the odd orange juice with a vodka.

During my treatment, and for some time after, I drank fresh juice every afternoon because I enjoyed it and it felt like a good thing to do. I always aimed to include vegetables of different colours in my cocktail – carrot, beetroot and something green such as celery, beetroot tops, spinach or even broccoli. I also added an apple or another piece of fruit to lighten the flavour.

There will always be people who argue against juice by pointing out that you need to eat the whole fruit or vegetable in order to get the full benefit, including fibre. I've no doubt that this is true but, during chemotherapy and radiotherapy, there was no way I could have eaten all of those raw vegetables every day. Juicing has to better than nothing at all as long as you enjoy the end result. While I like the taste, I can see that not everyone will get excited by the sight of a foaming, blood-red brew.

If you're not sure whether vegetable juice is for you, start slowly. Choose a fruit juice you like – apple is easy – and add a little carrot. If you enjoy that, gradually increase the quantity. You could then add a little beetroot and take it from there.

If you really can't bear the idea, forget it. No juice is worth making your life miserable over.

Fruit juice and medication

Recent research has suggested that fruit juice can interfere with certain medications. So far, grapefruit, orange and apple juices have been implicated; scientists are also warning that milk, tea and other beverages may have a similar effect. By contrast, another study found that cranberry juice may boost the effectiveness of chemotherapy used to treat ovarian cancer.

What to do?

Some scientists are suggesting that we should have four hours free from fruit juice each side of our medication. If you're taking tablets three or four times a day, that doesn't leave much of a window of opportunity, especially as no-one seems to be sure whether it's just juice you should avoid or the fruit itself. When other research is telling us that a diet rich in a variety of different fruits and vegetables could help reduce the risk of heart disease and some cancers, it's hard to know what to do for the best.

I now take my tablets with water rather than juice but haven't limited when I eat fruit. Is that reasonable? I've no idea – and I don't think anyone knows for sure. It's probably a question to raise with your doctor because advice might vary according to your particular medication.

Making it easy

It seems immensely unfair that it's much easier physically to eat badly than it is to eat well.

If you're feeling tired, unwell, miserable or just pressed for time, the effort involved in making a salad sandwich makes a biscuit or a bag of chips more appealing than ever. I found it helpful to keep a supply of healthy foods handy that are almost as fast and easy to prepare. Here are a few suggestions:

Toast or bread

Choose wholemeal if you like it, organic if possible. If you don't have much of an appetite, any bread can seem more tempting without the crusts. Try topping it with:

- peanut or other nut butter, with or without sliced banana
- tahini, a little cream cheese or ricotta or a scrape of butter with all-fruit jam
- tahini or avocado and tomato
- vegemite

Hommus, baba ghanoush or any other good-quality dip

These days even supermarkets sell ready-made dips without additives. Dip bread, toast, rice crackers, grissini or raw vegetables – just a washed carrot or celery stick will do.

Rice crackers – alone or with any easy topping.

Pretzels

Trail mix – dried fruit and nuts.

Left overs – even small amounts of carefully-stored left-over food can provide quick and tasty snacks.

A way of eating

Whether you're about to have surgery, coping with chemotherapy or radiotherapy or doing your best to stay well, it's good get into the habit of making each meal as nutritionally 'dense' as possible. That way, the odd indulgence is going to have a relatively small impact.

Where possible, steer away from special diet foods, 'lite' foods and anything heavily processed. Good, honest, high-quality foods provide the nutrients your body needs – fresh fruit and vegetables, meat and poultry that isn't loaded with fat and preservatives, fish, nuts, tofu, beans, pasta, grains, bread and olive oil.

For example, a bowl of muesli contains a wide range of vitamins, minerals, complex carbohydrates and protein – it's a great way to start the day.

Lunch and dinner should ideally include protein, complex carbohydrates and salad or vegetables. This could be anything from a salad sandwich to a pasta or rice dish or chicken or fish and salad with a bread roll.

Protein foods include tinned and fresh fish, lean meat, chicken, eggs and cheese. Vegans can use hommus, tofu, tempeh, nuts or nut spread. I quite like soy cheese, especially the cracked pepper version. It's nothing like real cheese, of course, but enjoyable in its own right.

Too much fat is not a good thing and it's important to remove the skin from chicken and cut visible fat from meat. However, that doesn't mean food has to be bland.

Normality at last!

A bonus for me when I started eating 'real' food was that it was so much more sustaining and satisfying. This helped me to normalise my eating and my weight.

For instance, rather than simply steaming your fish, poultry and meat, you could brown them in a tiny amount of olive oil in a non-stick pan, throw in some fresh or dried herbs then add a little water to finish off the cooking. The fat content is negligible, yet they're much more appetising. The same is true of vegetables.

Good food doesn't have to be boring or hard to cook. One of the most delicious meals I've eaten in a long time was pasta with a sauce made from onions and garlic, fresh tomatoes and fresh herbs which I made from scratch in about 15 minutes.

There are hundreds of cookery books filled with really delicious ideas for healthy food, and I've included some of my particular favourites on pages 143 – 155.

Water

For a long time, I drank nothing but coffee and alcohol with the occasional glass of orange juice. Water was not in my vocabulary. I also used to have a nagging headache on an almost permanent basis which became severe with monotonous regularity.

When I finally accepted that cup after cup of strong black coffee was doing little to help, I looked around for an alternative. Coffee substitutes did nothing for me, but I did find that I quite enjoyed many fruit and herb teas.

The headaches certainly improved, but it wasn't until I started drinking a couple of litres of water a day that they disappeared. I acquired this habit around the time of my operation, and I've rarely had to take a pain killer for a headache since.

It horrifies me now to think of how dehydrated I was for years of my life. Even when I was pregnant (and not drinking alcohol!) I used to pride myself on not needing to make those frequent dashes to the loo so many women complain about. I realise now that it was nothing to do with a strong bladder, I just wasn't drinking anything like as much fluid as I needed.

One downside of my first chemotherapy was it made water taste revolting – I simply couldn't drink it. Luckily, though, I could manage tangy fruit teas such as lemon, rosehip and blackcurrant. Fruit teas are also the only drinks I find palatable at room temperature, which meant I could make my drinks in a huge, 600ml mug, two tea bags at a time, then sip them through the day. Drinking too much too fast with the aim of 'getting it down' can make you feel just as nauseous as gulping too much food.

How much should we be drinking?

The amount of water we need to stay hydrated varies. An averagely-active person in a temperate climate will breathe, sweat and urinate away around 2.5 litres a day. Someone running a marathon in a hot, humid climate will need a lot more.

For years, the rule of thumb has been a daily intake of six to eight glasses of water on top of everything else we eat and drink. However, recent research suggests that water in fruit, vegetables, soup and juice *does* count towards the daily total. More surprisingly, it seems that water in tea and coffee can too. They were long thought to be diuretics – drinks which cause you to eliminate more water than you ingest – but now it appears they only behave like this when we drink them in large quantities.

Scientists are also warning us against taking drinking water to extremes. Some so-called 'detox' diets push the idea that swallowing huge quantities of water will 'flush out toxins'. That can sound very tempting, particularly when you're having chemotherapy, but too much water can be as dangerous as too little. Most health organisations advise against forcing yourself to drink or making yourself feel uncomfortable in any way.

10

EXERCISE

- Moving your arm
- Alleviate depression
- My routine

I used to say that I would only ever play a sport if I could hold a gin and tonic at the same time. I became very good at darts. I also bent my rule to include table soccer, pool and bar billiards. These may have demanded I put the gin and tonic (and the cigarette!) down between shots but at least I could play them in the pub.

It took me forty five years to get through the doors of a gym and, at the time of my diagnosis, I had been going reasonably regularly for two years.

I'm no convert to exercise – I hated every minute of the two or three pump classes I did each week. But I had reached the point of 'use it or lose it' when it came muscle tone and flexibility and I had promised myself I'd keep it up indefinitely.

The idea that I would have to stop because I had lost movement in my right arm depressed me. So I followed the exercises recommended in hospital to the letter and, less than a week after the operation, I could lift my arm straight above my head. Excellent – so that was that.

Unfortunately it hadn't occurred to me that, as wounds heal, tissue tends to tighten and contract. Day by day I was able to do less rather than more with my arm, or the same things hurt more, and I found that incredibly depressing. I felt doomed. I was failing. Despite doing everything I could I wasn't the perfect breast cancer patient.

Luckily, when the depression hit I was on holiday with a very wise and supportive friend. I also had time to persevere with the exercises twice a day – and no work to use as an excuse. By the end of the holiday I could feel that I was moving forward again, albeit frustratingly slowly. I had simply been too impatient and too ignorant of what was happening with my body.

I continued to exercise through chemotherapy and radiotherapy, gradually adding yoga moves and stretches my routine until I was exercising for around twenty minutes three or four times a week. My motivation was believing that the stronger my body, the more likely I was to cope with treatment for my disease. And it definitely helped with my self esteem. On the days I've exercised I generally feel better about myself, knowing I've done something positive towards becoming and staying healthy.

Over the years, my routine has changed a little in that the yoga I do for twenty minutes or so four or five times a week is a bit more strenuous. I still can't say I enjoy doing it, but I appreciate the effects too much to stop. The range of movement in my arms is just about indistinguishable, I'm as flexible as I was in my twenties and I think I'm stronger than I've ever been. I like that.

There's evidence now that exercising while you're being treated for cancer has a number of different benefits. Interestingly, these include a reduction in fatigue and an increase in stamina as well as increased strength, better sleep and even reduced nausea. Exercise is also important

---

Your best is always good enough

Overcoming the temptation to say 'if I can't be perfect, I won't bother at all' is a continuing challenge for me. It's a dangerous attitude which I believe is subtly encouraged by a lot that we read and hear. I think we all need to tell ourselves a hundred times a day that doing the best we can in whatever circumstances we find ourselves is always good enough.

---

in terms of emotional strength. It can help alleviate depression though, ironically, there's little more difficult than motivating yourself to do anything at all when a black mood sets in.

If you can just take that initial step, there's a good chance that you will end up feeling better. But, knowing that, there used to be mornings when I simply couldn't manage it. These were the days when I leant especially hard on the techniques I talk about in Chapter 12.

Choosing your time

While I was being treated, my children were old enough to understand 'keep out', and I found that the best time for me to exercise was the minute I got out of bed. If you have younger children, you may feel there's no such thing as a best time.

You could try making your exercise the first thing you do when your baby or toddler falls asleep. You could sit them in front of a favourite DVD. Or you may have to wait until they've gone to bed though, by then, you may feel close to collapsing yourself.

Bear in mind that watching you exercise could provide entertainment in itself. Your children may be sufficiently interested to sit and watch, or even join in.

Some exercises that have worked for me

My aim is always to be flexible, with a strong back and stomach, not-too-saggy bottom and as little as possible flapping under my arms. I also like to keep working my arms and shoulders so that they stay flexible. This sequence below covers off all the basics for me, but there are many other alternatives.

As with any form of exercise, it's important to check with your doctor that these exercises are right for you. And always stay within a range of movement and effort that feels comfortable for you – never push yourself too hard.

1.   Neck stretch

Standing comfortably, let your head drop forward towards your chest. Bring it up and tilt it towards your right shoulder. Bring it up and drop it back. Bring it up and tilt it towards your left shoulder. Be gentle, but be sure to feel a stretch.

2. Shoulder stretch

Stand with your feet shoulder width apart and clasp your hands behind your back, palms up. Bend forward from the waist, letting your arms follow the movement, until you feel a good stretch in your back and shoulders.

3. Shoulder rolls

Stand comfortably with your arms hanging loosely at your sides. Lift one shoulder as high as you can then slowly rotate it, making the movement as big as you can. Repeat in the opposite direction, and then with the opposite shoulder.

4. Cat stretch

Kneel down with your arms straight beneath your shoulders and your knees directly beneath your hips. Arch your back, pushing up between your shoulder blades and tilting your pelvis forward slightly so that you're really hollowing out your stomach as you draw it towards your spine. Slowly return to your starting position and continue through, moving your pelvis back and lifting your chest so your back is hollowed out in the other direction. Look up but not too high – don't strain your neck. Repeat a few times, slowly and in a controlled way.

5. Back release

I've heard more than one back expert say that, if we did nothing but this exercise a few times a day, we'd be much less likely to suffer from back pain.

Lie on your back with your knees bent and your feet together and close to your buttocks. Have your hands clasped behind your head or stretched out to the side. Keeping your knees together gradually lower them to the right as you turn to look the opposite way, keeping the movement controlled and only taking them as far as you can until your shoulder starts to lift. Repeat to the left, again turning your head to look the other way.

6. Sit ups

Lie on the floor with your knees bent and your hands behind your head for support. Keeping the small of your back on the floor, and without craning your head forward, tighten your stomach muscles and curl your shoulders off the floor. At first, this could be a tiny movement. Even when your muscles are strong you should probably limit your lift to an angle of 40 degrees or so.

If you want, you can add a few extra sit-ups with a twist to one side and then the other. This will strengthen the muscles along the sides of your stomach and help define your waist.

7. Arm builders

Use any light weight for added resistance – for instance, a small water bottle containing as much water as feels comfortable. Don't ever struggle to lift more weight than feels easy for you.

- *Biceps (at the front of your upper arms)*

Stand with your arms at your sides, palms forward. Lift the weight as far as you can without moving anything other than the forearm.

- *Triceps (at the back of your upper arms)*

Lift one arm straight above your head. Raise and lower your hand, keeping your upper arm very still and close to your ear.

This is not an easy exercise to do unless you have regained full flexibility in your arm and shoulder. However, I like it because the other easy at-home triceps exercises I've found involve working against your own body weight, which might be too much for women who are at risk from lymphoedema.

8. Lunges

Take a big step forward with your right leg and bend your knees, keeping your back straight. Stop just before your left knee touches the floor. Tighten your bottom and push up again. Don't push yourself too hard – lunges and the squats which follow can be very tiring. If it all feels too much, just go for a walk or even walk on the spot for a couple of minutes.

9. Squats

Stand in front of, and close to, a straight-backed chair. Lower yourself gently, as if you were going to sit down, then tighten your bottom and push up back to standing before you do.

10. The tower

I've included this exercise because it's one I struggled with for weeks, never quite being able to straighten my right arm. When I finally did, I felt triumphant – as if the last hurdle had been crossed – and I still do it regularly, even at my computer, mostly because I can!

Standing comfortably, feet apart, place your hands over your head and interlink your fingers, palms up. Stretch your arms up as high as you can, getting your elbows as close to locked as possible. Repeat with your hand clasped the opposite way – the other thumb on top.

11

MEDITATION

- **The benefits of meditation**
- **Getting started**
- **Techniques to try**

Meditation can represent anything from a profound religious or spiritual experience to a way of unwinding after a hard day.

When I first started to hear about the health benefits associated with meditation I was very excited. Unfortunately my excitement lasted for about two minutes flat – as long as it took to read the recommendation that I meditate for 30-40 minutes three or more times a day.

Meditation was a regular feature in the books I read about healing, but they all left me with the feeling that it must be taken very seriously, taking up far more time than I could ever hope to spare. I decided that the best thing to do was forget about it.

It was a few weeks before I came back to meditation with a more open mind. I had had a few sessions of hypnotherapy and was starting to appreciate the joy of deep relaxation. I could see that meditation might be a way of recreating that sensation at home, even if I only did it occasionally. I was also starting to believe that meditation really might be a way to counterbalance the inevitable worries, stress and tension we experience every day.

There is evidence that meditation can decrease heart and respiration rates and help the brain achieve a state of 'restful alertness'. Meditation can also help you feel less anxious and more in control, and ease depression. Some people will develop heightened self-awareness, personal insight and self-understanding – a feeling of being more at peace with themselves. It has to be worth a try!

When I noticed that the two hospitals where I was receiving treatment both recommended meditation classes for patients with cancer I decided that I couldn't afford to ignore it any longer.

Practice

I quickly discovered that meditation is both incredibly easy and frustratingly difficult. It's so easy that we do it unconsciously – if you have ever found yourself 'miles away' while staring into a crackling fire, listening to music or gazing out on to a beautiful landscape, you have meditated. For a few moments your brain was empty of all thought and filled with stillness and tranquility – just what you hope to achieve with meditation.

On the other hand, when you set about consciously regaining the same state, it can seem impossible. In reality it could take years of practice before you can slip into a meditative state at will but this really doesn't matter.

The very essence of meditation is learning to accept things as they are, including your own 'performance'. There's no need to judge yourself, though this is a difficult concept in itself when most of us have grown up in a world which tends to value competitiveness. When I tried to meditate a couple of times and 'failed', I had to fight hard to suppress my instinct to stop trying.

I am still doing some kind of meditation on a reasonably regular basis. I have managed to get beyond the initial stages to a more profound and restful silence on my own only a few times – I find it easier to use guided meditation. What I can definitely do is benefit from 20 minutes or so of physical relaxation every night. That in itself is very worthwhile.

How do you start?

There are many ways to meditate, ranging from sitting still to walking, the whirling of the Dervishes and the so-called chaotic meditation of the Rajneesh. They all have the intention of quietening the busy mind. For most of us, though, sitting still is the most practical way to start.

For this, there are a few basic requirements.

A *quiet place*

That means somewhere you won't be disturbed by people or the phone. If you have young children, it will almost certainly mean waiting until they are out of the house or asleep.

A *comfortable or poised posture*

From the full and half lotus to the kneeling stance of Christian prayer, most traditional poses fulfil two important functions – they keep the body in balance by maintaining a straight spine and they stop you from falling asleep. I'm sure the lotus positions are wonderful if you can manage them. If you can't, you can try sitting on a cushion with your legs stretched out in front of you, on a straight-backed chair with your feet flat on the floor, or in any other position that is comfortable for you. In each case, let your hands rest loosely in your lap.

Lying down is not recommended for meditation because you are so likely to fall asleep. However, it's the position I use most frequently.

I meditate in bed, either first thing in the morning, when I very rarely fall asleep, or last thing at night, when I sometimes do. Even then, I seem to enjoy a particularly restful night, which is good in itself.

A relaxed body

The first step to meditation is a relaxed body.

Progressive relaxation is genuinely very easy – you simply relax each muscle group in turn.

If you're working from your toes to your head, the sequence might be feet, calves, thighs, buttocks, stomach, back, chest, hands, arms, shoulders, neck, scalp, jaw, tongue, eyes and forehead. Alternatively, you can start with the forehead and work down.

If you find it hard to isolate different muscle groups, or to know for sure whether your muscles are fully relaxed, tense them before you try to relax. This makes it much easier to feel the difference.

Another progressive relaxation is to focus on tension in specific areas as you breathe in, then release the tension as you breathe out. Again you can move up from your toes or down from your forehead.

Meditation techniques to try

Meditating on the breath

A way described as one of the simplest is to sit quietly and focus on your breathing. Theoretically, your mind will gradually become absorbed in the rhythm of inhalation and exhalation. Your breathing will become slower and deeper; your mind will become more tranquil and aware.

In reality, you will barely have taken your first breath before you find yourself thinking about what to cook for tomorrow's dinner, when your next chemotherapy treatment is due or an whether you turned off the iron. This is totally normal. Each time your mind wanders, simply acknowledge the thought and gently bring your focus back to your breathing.

Try not to feel frustrated or dissatisfied – the idea is not to judge your performance. Just believe that, the more you practice, the longer you will find yourself able to meditate between intruding thoughts. And remember that any approximation of meditation is better than no meditation at all.

Meditating on a sound

A word like 'peace' or 'God', or a syllable like 'om' repeated silently with each outgoing breath could provide a stronger focus. As with meditating on the breath, your concentration is likely to wander quickly at first. Again, each time bring your mind gently back to your word or syllable.

Acknowledging your thoughts

Another way of approaching meditation is to imagine that your thoughts are like clouds drifting across the sky. As they slip into your consciousness, simply acknowledge them and let them pass or dissolve. Gradually, there will be fewer clouds to interrupt your meditation.

Guided meditation

There are hundreds of CDs and tapes offering guided meditation and creative visualisation. I have tried a few and I found that the first thing to look for is a voice that doesn't become distracting in itself. This, of course, is a very personal thing, so don't give up if the first one you listen to grates rather than soothes.

Come back gently to the world

Whichever technique you choose, when you have finished meditating, sit quietly for a few minutes with your eyes closed, then open them and begin to move and stretch your muscles. Wriggle your fingers and toes, and wait a couple of minutes before you stand up.

Mindfulness

Mindfulness is a slightly different approach to meditation because, rather than being something you do at particular times, it means being fully aware of whatever you're doing in any particular moment.

A simple mindfulness exercise is to make use of all of your senses, becoming conscious of everything you can see, hear, feel externally, feel internally and smell.

I do this as often as I remember, but particularly when I'm outdoors. I find it transforms even something as simple as a trip to the corner shop. In the past, I would have marched up the road totally preoccupied with my thoughts and worries. If I was aware of the walk at all it would be to resent it for taking up so much time! Now I consciously take notice of everything around me – trees, sky, the sounds of the birds...even things like the noise my feet are making and how my clothes feel against my skin. This is being 'in the moment' and it's often a surprisingly pleasant place to be. For me, being more mindful has opened up many opportunities for joy that I had overlooked every day. It has also helped me to focus more on appreciating the things I do have in my life than fretting about the things I don't.

Another interesting time to practice mindfulness is when you're eating. If you read Chapter 9, you may remember that I talked about tasting and relishing every mouthful of your favourite food. This is actually being mindful, and it creates a very different experience from the usual one of eating while we're having a chat, watching TV or reading a book.

If any of this interests you, you might want to look up Jon Kabat-Zinn. He is probably the best known exponent of mindfulness and, as Professor of Medicine emeritus at the University of Massachusetts Medical School, he has done much to introduce its benefits to the mainstream.

Something for everyone

Meditation has evolved from many different religions and philosophies, so this list is far from exhaustive. If you're interested in looking at other techniques you will find plenty of information on the Internet or at your local library. As with anything unfamiliar, be sure to do your research before making any sort of commitment, particularly if that means spending a lot of money.

12

HELPING YOURSELF
TO FEEL BETTER

- A new way of thinking
- A more positive frame of mind
- Choosing your future
- Your point of power is now

It sounds logical to expect that everyday problems will pale into insignificance when cancer comes into your life. This may be true of the minor ones – whether to holiday in Australia or overseas, whether your child should learn violin or piano – but, unfortunately, the big ones can be stubbornly persistent.

Once the news that I had cancer had sunk in I thought I would start to see life differently. I waited for colours to look brighter, flowers to smell sweeter and my troubles to fade into the background as I suddenly started to cherish every second I was alive.

It didn't happen.

At the time I was a single mother with four children aged between nine and 16. Two of them had major and ongoing health problems.

As my ex-husband helped me to run my business I had six people to support, yet my finances were totally out of control. I had debts, no assets and a mounting tax problem. As I was freelance, my income was unpredictable and I was living from cheque to cheque, constantly having to chase money to pay my bills.

I'm sure I don't need to mention that I had no trauma or income protection insurance.

I was living in a rented house, and this was in an area I hated. My home was in a constant state of chaos. I seemed to do be doing nothing but lurch from crisis to crisis. Cancer felt like the final straw.

It didn't help that I kept on hearing about the power of a positive attitude to help me to feel better, and perhaps even to get better. Where was someone who had been struggling with depression for years, and who was already taking antidepressants, going to find the right state of mind for coping with cancer?

Getting my head around a new way of thinking

When I began my search, I thought I might not make it past the starting gate. The phrase 'positive thinking' scared me because I believed it could mean only one of two things, neither of which had a chance of working for me.

1. Another way of saying 'count your blessings' or 'there's always someone worse off than you'. Of course my heart goes out to people in countries ripped apart by war and famine or who are suffering in other unspeakable ways, but that didn't change the fact that I had breast cancer, or make me feel any better about myself.

2. The attitude expounded by some motivational speakers – the ones who assume that your goal is to be an Olympic athlete or head of a multinational corporation. While I admire the entrepreneur who works 18 hours a day in

order to get his business up and running, or the swimmer who gets up at 4am every day in order to practice for four hours before going off to work or school, these people have nothing to do with me – they could be from another planet. Rather than inspire me, thoughts of their achievements would leave me feeling even more inadequate when I was struggling to find the energy to walk round the block with my dogs.

The temptation was to give up and accept that life's a bitch and then you die. Only the thought of my children drove me to find ways of making myself feel better.

What I found was very interesting. Not only did I cope with breast cancer, I also started to cope with problems that had dogged me for most of my life.

Turning my life around

A friend had recommended I see a hypnotherapist who is also a spiritual and emotional counsellor. I went along because I was looking for anything that might help reduce my exploding stress levels. It did. But, far more importantly, I got my first glimpse of the path that would turn my life around – the idea that I could control my life by changing the way I think.

At first I was cynical. It sounded a bit too 'new age' and alternative for my liking. I also found it hard to believe that where I was now was the result of my own thinking rather than things that were out of my control.

I bought a couple of books that had similar messages, looked up a few sites on the Internet and spoke to friends who are doctors. I was surprised to discover that there is now medical support for the belief that a thought is much more powerful than I had ever imagined.

For instance, the placebo effect is accepted as fact by the medical profession. As long as someone believes he or she is taking medication, a sugar pill will often have the same effect as the real thing.

Research has also shown that thinking alters the biochemistry of the brain; there's even a scientific discipline called psychoneuroimmunology – the study of how chemical messengers released as part of the thought process have a physical effect on the body.

And then there's psychosomatic illness. I have had first hand experience of this phenomenon, something else that is accepted as fact by the medical profession. If it's possible to think yourself ill and miserable , then might it not just be possible to think ourselves well and happy?

This is all food for thought but, for me, it isn't the most important point. Whether or not a positive attitude has any effect on how long we survive, it will profoundly affect the quality of our lives.

When I was first diagnosed with breast cancer I was angry, short-tempered and sorry for myself. My thoughts looped endlessly through 'I can't cope. I can't die because of my children. But I can't cope.' And, of course, I knew I was making everyone else's lives as miserable as my own so I was permanently racked with guilt.

When I learned to think more positively, everything changed. How I felt about myself, how I viewed every day, my relationship with my children, the atmosphere at home.

Of course there were times when I felt sad or depressed or afraid or overwhelmed and there's absolutely nothing wrong with this. Another misconception about positive thinking is that it means feeling happy all the time. This is a terrible pressure to place on someone who is trying to cope with cancer. No-one can be happy all the time and, if you believe you should be, you are opening the door to feelings of failure – of not being good enough, not wanting to live enough, not caring about your family enough…feelings that will lead to even greater despair.

Staying positive isn't struggling to deny what you feel in order to change something in the future. I believe that staying positive means accepting what you feel and making choices that will help you to feel better every day.

What do you really want?

I decided to keep my second appointment with my counsellor and to do my homework. This was to think about the things I really wanted from life – things that would genuinely make me happier – and write them down in the present tense.

I quickly discovered that this isn't as easy as it sounds.

We may think we want things because other people told us we should – 'you should get a better job', 'you should lose weight', 'you should settle down'. We may think we want things because they're what other people have, or because they're things we think we should have in order to appear successful.

When I first wrote down what I wanted from life I included a relationship. But, the more I thought about it, the more I realised that I simply didn't have room in my life for a new man at that time. In fact, a new relationship would have almost certainly exacerbated many of the issues

I was working to resolve. The only reason I thought I wanted a relationship was because some well-meaning friends were telling me it was just what I needed – that it would be good for me. As soon as I dropped the idea I experienced a huge surge of relief.

In Xandria Williams' book *Beating the Blues* she talks about scripting – writing a script of your life is if it were already exactly the way you want it to be. This concept worked brilliantly for me. As soon as I started writing, the things that really mattered to me began to click into focus – and they weren't always what I would have expected.

I find scripting easy and very exciting, but that may be because I've been a writer for so long. If you find it hard to get started, here are some points you may want to cover.

- What is the date – how far are you in the future?
- Where are you living?
- If you're working, what job are you doing?
- What is happening in your family life?
- What are you doing to help others?
- How did you get to where you are?

Your scenario needs to be optimistic, but also realistic. 'I am living in a mansion bought with sponsorship money I received following my Olympic gold medal win in the 100 metres freestyle' is probably a bit too ambitious for anyone over the age of 12. 'I am living in a mansion bought with my lotto win' is out of your control.

Try to include enough detail in your script to bring it to life. When you've finished you should be able to visualise yourself in the situation you have created and feel excited by it. If some parts are a bit woolly, it could be that

My script

It is (date). I am sitting in a beautiful green and shady space, reflecting on my wonderful life and how perfectly everything is unfolding.

I have a home I love in a place I love, with plenty of space for me and room for my children to live or stay in comfort. I love my work as an author, coach and speaker and appreciate having an opportunity make a positive difference in people's lives. I have a rich social life, good friends and happy relationships with my children.

I am profoundly grateful for my vibrant health, my happiness, all of the love in my life and my financial security; for having the freedom to live my life to the full and to share my abundance.

you don't really want them to be included. Try the vision without them – and keep an open mind. It may take a few days of fiddling to get your script to a stage where you feel completely happy and comfortable with it. When you have, the things you really want should be much more clear.

Using my script as a prompt, I then wrote down the things I really wanted in life – again in the present tense.

1. I am vibrantly healthy.
2. I am wealthy and in control of my finances.
3. I am a successful author.
4. I am living in a beautiful, spacious and tidy home with a wonderful outlook.
5. I am tranquil and happy.
6. I love, respect and approve of myself.
7. I am the mother of happy children.

My counsellor explained that these were my affirmations, and that I was to repeat them out loud at least once a day and to myself as often as I could bear. But first she said I should remove number seven. However desperately I want my children to be happy they can only achieve happiness for themselves. Oh well.

At first I felt ridiculous – it was so patently obvious that I was not all I was claiming to be that I might as well have been chanting 'I am a three-legged turtle'. Even worse, the affirmations kept on reminding me of how much of a failure I felt when I compared my reality with an ideal I believed I could never achieve.

Then the remarkable happened. One day it occurred to me that they were no longer totally preposterous. Without consciously doing anything in particular, I had started to make decisions which were bringing my life closer to where I wanted it to be.

Affirmation 1. I am vibrantly healthy

At the time of my 'enlightenment' I had completed one 12-week cycle of chemotherapy, was in the middle of six weeks of radiotherapy and had another 12-week cycle of chemotherapy to go – yet I felt fantastic. People who hadn't seen me for a while said I looked better than I had before cancer. More than one told me I had the positive glow of an athlete! By eating well, exercising and meditating I was helping to create the vibrant health I wanted.

Affirmation 2. I am wealthy and in control of my finances

When I was growing up, my mother lived on a widow's pension and the little she earned as a clerk while I was at school. We were not well off and, when her long-standing illness became more debilitating, we became poorer. Yet she never failed to pay a bill on time.

There was a row of jars in the larder labelled 'electricity', 'gas', 'hire purchase', 'food', 'clothes', 'holidays' and probably a couple more I can't remember. Each week she would allocate her money according to a precise budget. She never, ever borrowed from one to pay another. In fact, apart from the carefully-controlled hire purchase of the occasional household item, she never borrowed at all.

As a child, I followed her example, religiously saving my pocket money and putting money aside for special occasions. Then, when I went to university, I quickly fell into the pattern that was to determine my financial life for the next 30 years – spend first, worry later.

I've done a lot of worrying.

For as long as I can remember, everything I have done in life has been coloured by debt and lack of money. Yet I have consistently earned a good salary as a copywriter and journalist.

My excuse to myself was that I was too 'creative' to worry about my finances. Accountants weren't expected to be writers, so why should I have to think like an accountant? I told myself that I couldn't be bothered with financial control – that was for other people. Yet, in my script, I was financially secure. I couldn't deny any longer how important this was to me.

On the surface, things looked pretty much the same. I was still looking back on three years of tax chaos. I was still struggling to pay my bills. But there was a big difference – my attitude had changed

It was as if I had drawn a line beneath the years of disaster and was starting afresh, even though I had a huge job ahead to resolve my problems. I had started to put money aside and think twice about everything I spent. I had also put an efficient filing system in place for the first time in years.

I certainly wasn't wealthy, but I had at least acknowledged my need for control and was taking steps towards achieving it.

Affirmation 3. I am a successful author

I had finally started the book I had been thinking about for months and was working on it almost every day.

Affirmation 4. I am living in a beautiful, spacious and tidy home with a wonderful outlook

Mess had been a major issue throughout my adult life, and the main bone of contention throughout my marriage. My ex-husband and I were truly the second Odd Couple – he the living, breathing expression of the term 'anal retentive' while my total disregard for order would have tried the patience of Oscar Madison himself.

Over the years I had justified my domestic chaos in much the same way as I justified my financial chaos – I believed it wasn't important to me. I also had a chip on my shoulder about renting my home. I told myself that there was no point in bothering with my environment until I owned my own house.

Once again my script had shown me otherwise. A pleasant environment mattered to me, and I had set about achieving it.

Within two weeks, I had filled the garage twice over with things I didn't need. I've no idea where all of the rubbish came from. But, by removing it, I had made my home if not exactly beautiful, then a lot more beautiful than it used to be – and it certainly felt a lot more spacious. It was also much more tidy. As for the wonderful outlook, I had at least removed the broken pot with the dead jasmine plant from outside my front door!

I am tranquil and happy

Happiness hasn't always featured strongly in my vocabulary. I have a long history of depression, with the whole of my twenties dominated by bulimia, alcoholism, depression and suicide attempts. I had been taking antidepressants for most of my adult life.

When I went into hospital for my mastectomy I forgot to take the antidepressants with me and, even nine years on, I haven't taken one since.

As I said earlier, I had times when I felt worried, sad, frightened and overwhelmed. My cancer didn't stop other crises in their tracks. But, thanks to progress of my other affirmations, I was feeling less stressed, more calm and something as close to happy as I'd ever felt in my life.

Even my children commented on the 'new me' – they told me I was more fun and easier to be around.

I love, respect and approve of myself

Eating well and exercising, gaining control over money, writing my book, keeping my home tidier – every step I took towards what I really wanted in my life made me feel better about myself. I was starting to approve of the things I did every day instead of hating myself for being a failure.

Carving a new path

Looking back, it all sounds stupidly simple. I had written down what I wanted and then taken action to make it happen. But, if it were so simple, why hadn't I done it years ago?

I believe that I had spent my life subconsciously sabotaging my own happiness. The excuses were all in place – 'not important to me', 'too busy', 'not successful enough' – and I had been acting on them for years.

My affirmations had alerted me to what really did matter in my life. Repeating them regularly was somehow reprogramming my subconscious to believe that they were true. And, because I was starting to believe that they were true, I was also starting to *act* as if they were true. Imagine, for instance, that I receive an ominous-looking letter from the tax department. If I subconsciously believe that I financial control doesn't matter to me, I'll do exactly what I've done for years – throw it into the back of a drawer and pretend it doesn't exist. On the other hand, if I subconsciously believe that I am in control of my finances, I will open the letter, read it and deal with it as best I can.

The table opposite shows other examples that work in the same way.

It's easy to see how, once the thinking changes, the affirmations become self-fulfilling prophecies. If found this a very inspirational thought – I had always assumed that the only spirals were downward!

Old belief	Action	New belief	Action
I'm very unwell.	No action – ill people don't move around too much.	I'm vibrantly healthy.	I exercise regularly and eat well.
I live in a messy home	I don't see or register the clutter around me.	I live in a tidy home	I not only see the clutter I move it.
I am stressed and stretched to my limit by the disasters that keep befalling me.	It seems only natural that I would lose my temper easily and snap at my children.	I am happy and tranquil and take everything calmly in my stride	I have more patience and am slower to lose my temper.
I'm not good enough to be a successful author.	I avoid putting myself to the test by never finishing anything.	I am a successful author.	I write regularly, finish my book and do my best to promote it.

Looking for causes

I was in my twenties when my depression was at its most extreme, and this coincided with studying psychology at university. Between my studies and seeing a psychiatrist I managed to become totally self-absorbed and, worse still,

> The idea of mind power is old news to most athletes. They take it for granted that affirmations and visualisations will form an integral part of their training.

locked into analysing and re-analysing the past that I blamed for all of my problems. I had plenty of material to work with. I'm still convinced, for instance, that my alcoholism and bulimia were fuelled by insecurity.

When my father died after months of being in hospital, it was at a time when people really believed that a three-year-old could have no concept of death. They genuinely thought that the best way to help me was to say nothing. So no-one told me what had happened to him – and the wall of silence was so effective that I knew I must never ask.

It was three or four years before I discovered the truth, and then in the most unlikely way. A teacher asked me why I was paying for school lunches. She told me they should be free, adding "Your father is dead, isn't he?" That was the first I'd heard about it – and, even then, I didn't dare raise the subject with my mother.

Soon after, she was admitted to hospital for the first of several long stays. Children were not allowed to visit, and, perhaps because she was critically ill for a while, once again everyone thought it best to tell me nothing. For eight weeks I had no idea whether I would ever see her again.

I know that this secrecy was intended to protect me – but I also have no doubt that this 'abandonment' caused profound damage to my subconscious mind.

Unfortunately, it was another forty or so years before I realised that this didn't mean I had no choice but to suffer dire consequences for the rest of my life.

Forget the past!

The reason I felt so doomed was that understanding and discussing the causes of my problems made absolutely no difference to the way I felt.

The beauty of my new approach is that I have been able to move on. I have come to believe that the point of power really is now – things can start to change from this very moment.

Knowing that I no longer needed to rake over the past in the hope of improving the future gave me a wonderful feeling of liberation. However, this didn't mean I could simply hammer a lid on my past.

In order to move forward we need to be able to release the past and I had some difficult issues I had to confront before I could do this. I could only manage this with the help of my counsellor. If you're in a similar situation, I strongly recommend that you get help too.

Whether this is a psychologist, an experienced counsellor or a more alternative practitioner, I suggest you try to find someone who comes with a personal recommendation. Even then, if you don't feel comfortable with the person, try someone else. You must feel that the person you're talking to is empathetic and on your wavelength otherwise it will be even more difficult to speak with the honesty you need.

It's interesting to look back on childhood and to consider the influences that helped to shape us. But, unless we let go of those influences, we will continue to feel as helpless and out of control as we did when we were small.

As adults, we have to believe that we have the power and the freedom to make choices. I found the concept both exhilarating and terrifying – it means I have nothing to hide behind or blame any more. It also means that I have no limitations.

GOAL SETTING FOR PEOPLE WHO DON'T SET GOALS

- **Let's be realistic…**
- **Goals for every day**
- **Goals you can't fail to achieve**

As an advertising copywriter, I had been writing about setting and achieving financial goals for years. I had also come across goal setting as recommended by motivational and personal development speakers.

Obviously, I had been impervious to my own wisdom as far as the financial goals were concerned. I had also actively avoided setting any personal development goals. This was because the books and tapes my ex-husband felt he ought to buy and then left lying around frightened me half to death. (Unfortunately, they also had the same effect on him.)

This is not because they're bad – it's just that they are aimed at people who are very different from me.

As an example, I was recently listening to a live recording of an Anthony Robbins seminar. One of the stories he told to illustrate the value of persistence was about Colonel Sanders, founder of Kentucky Fried Chicken. Apparently, the Colonel took his recipe to 1,009 restaurants before he found someone interested enough to give his idea a try. Robbins asked his audience how many of them would

Is it worth it?

Soon after I was diagnosed, I mentioned to friends that I planned to give up advertising so that I could concentrate on writing books. At first I was puzzled by their reaction – they were so very impressed that I was thinking about a change of career. Then it dawned on me. I was making plans for a future they thought I might not have.

When you have cancer, it's easy to feel despondent about goal setting. At first I found myself thinking twice about buying a new pair of boots, let alone planning my next summer holiday!

The fact is I might die before all of my goals are fulfilled. It may be from cancer or I may be hit by that proverbial bus – either way, I would hardly regret the work I have done in trying to achieve all the things I want most from life.

Goals aren't just about the future. Travelling towards them can help us to feel better every day.

have given up after 500 people? All but two people said yes, they would have given up after 500 tries. The others said they would have kept on trying.

Had I been entrusted with the recipe for fried chicken, I wouldn't have approached a single restaurant owner in person. I would have sent letter. Maybe 20 letters. Then I would have given up.

That's the way I am. I don't consider that there's anything particularly wrong with me. And there's certainly nothing wrong with Anthony Robbins – he has inspired countless people to enjoy more fulfilling and successful lives. It's just that I don't feel I'd make his starting line.

With this history, I was surprised to realise that I had already started to set and achieve goals. My affirmations were goals for future happiness, and I was already taking action towards them.

The difference was that now I had my subconscious working for me rather than against me. At last I was beginning to see how goals setting worked for other people – and see how it could work for me by providing concrete support for my affirmations.

The Domini Stuart approach to goal setting

1. Set your goal

If you have established your affirmations the hard work is over – your goals are clear, specific and realistic.

2. Write down a series of achievable steps that will take you directly to each goal

The key to success is knowing that each step is achievable before you write it down. For instance, in making 'I am vibrantly healthy' a goal as well as a affirmation, my steps included:

- Take vitamins every day
- Eat mostly organic food
- Walk the dogs every day
- Exercise three times a week
- Enjoy one or two cups of coffee a day
- Enjoy one glass of wine a day, two on special occasions
- Meditate five times a week

These are things I feel confident that I can achieve. In the past I would have felt compelled to aim higher, including steps like 'stop drinking completely', 'never eat chocolate again', 'get up at 5.30 every morning and go for a run'. These would be doomed to failure – probably on the first day – and I would have been plunged into an even deeper depression.

If you find there isn't a series of achievable steps to your goal, your goal is unrealistic. For instance, if you make your goal 'to win Lotto' there's nothing you can do but by a ticket and hope. This isn't a goal, it's a wish. In other cases, you may not need to abandon your goal completely. Try playing around with it for a while to see if you can find a way of putting manageable steps in place.

3. Write a realistic deadline next to each step

Again, 'realistic' is the key. If you earn $500 a week, there's no way you're going to have saved $5,000 for a holiday in three months unless you can create another source of income.

4. Achieve your goal

You know that each step is achievable within the deadline, so you know you can't fail. All you have to do is take action.

You're sure to come across an obstacle from time to time. Rise to the challenge by changing your thinking or your approach. Be creative. Imagine what someone you admire would do in the circumstances. You may need to create a detour with a few more steps than you were expecting. This doesn't matter as long as you adjust your deadlines accordingly, keep your final goal in mind and persist with your journey.

As motivational speaker Zig Zigglar once said, failure is the route of least persistence! (Within reason, of course!)

Visualise achieving your goals

I like to bring my goals to life by seeing myself on a journey to success.

I imagine that I'm standing at one station and my goal is waiting at another. Each step is then a station in between. As long as each step is achievable, all I have to do is get on the train and keep on travelling!

Can a man be a goal?

If you are aiming for a fulfilling new relationship it isn't possible to have quite as much control over your steps as when you're, say, planning to move house, but that doesn't mean you can't have this as a goal.

First, you need to be sure that your subconscious is working for you as effectively as it can. Check your affirmation and make sure that it's not too specific. From the purely physical point of view, for instance, it would be better to say 'I am seeing a man whom I find very attractive' than 'I am going out with a tall, slim, dark-haired man with blue eyes'. It would be a pity if your subconscious failed to register your ideal partner because he didn't match up to your imagined ideal.

You also need to think about ways in which you might meet this person. If you keep on doing the same thing you're going to keep on seeing the same people, so be ready to accept all invitations and try out some new destinations. More women are giving Internet dating sites a try. These are all the kinds of activities which will form your 'stations'.

Either way, try not to focus too strongly on the soul mate aspect. If you enjoy pottery but the man of your dreams isn't taking the same class, don't feel you have to flit from interest to interest in an attempt to find him. Many people meet their perfect partner through friends and a group of people who share an interest with you offers great potential for establishing new friendships.

14

WHEN THINGS GO WRONG

- No-one's life is perfect
- Fighting off depression
- Getting back in control

The idea that you can think yourself into feeling better and creating the life you want for yourself is incredibly empowering – most of the time. But what about when things are going wrong?

When I was first starting to believe I had the power to forge a better future, bouts of anxiety or depression became doubly stressful. The bad feeling associated with the emotion itself was compounded by the fear that I was failing to maintain the 'correct' frame of mind. The pressure to stay positive and cheerful was almost unbearable.

It took me a while – and my counsellor's help – to accept that there's a difference between having a good attitude and being happy all the time.

No-one's life is endlessly perfect. We are all bound to feel fear, anxiety and stress and only the certifiably insane would laugh and smile their way through disappointment, money worries, children's problems, emotional trauma or any other of the issues that inevitably arise in our lives from time to time.

We have to accept that there are some events we simply can't control. However, we can choose how we react to them. We can't stop it from being our birthday, but we can choose whether to look forward to a great opportunity for a happy celebration or sink into depression because we're a year older.

Putting it all to the test

Towards the end of my treatment, external factors beyond my control were starting to make me feel overwhelmed again. I found myself slipping back into my old ways.

I had gradually stopped all of my exercising apart from short walks with the dogs. I was once again falling asleep on the sofa at 10 o'clock, waking at midnight and watching bad TV until three or even four in the morning. I was then going to bed and meditating occasionally, but generally falling asleep too quickly to reap the benefits. The house was starting to look untidy. Some nights I fell asleep without working on my book at all.

This was a familiar place – and a place I really didn't want to be.

Depression was setting in, and depression is the enemy of action. Lack of action also tends to feed off itself. Once you stop doing one thing it's suddenly a lot easier to stop doing another.

On the upside, action – even on a small scale – can help pull you out of a dark period. The problem is that, when you're depressed, motivation is hard to find.

The answer for me was to lower my expectations even further – to find anything, however small, that I knew I could achieve. Taking action of any kind helped me reverse the downward spiral I was experiencing and get me back on track for what I really wanted to do.

1. Make a list of everything you could possibly do which would make you feel better about yourself. No action is too small. If you're depressed, you might be finding it hard to get out of bed in the morning. Giving yourself a definite time to get up and then deciding to shower and dress immediately rather than sit around in your dressing gown could be the place to get started. If this is not a problem for you, it may be starting the day with a healthy breakfast. Bothering to make vegetable juice for yourself. Going for a walk. Anything you're not doing now that you wish you were. Make your action specific and measurable – it has to be something you can tick off at the end of the day.

2. Choose the easiest thing on your list.

3. Do it as soon as you can, cross it off your list and then forget about your list for the rest of the day.

4. The following day, if you feel up to it, do the two easiest things from your list. If you don't, just repeat the thing you did the day before. If that was a one-off, choose the next easiest thing.

5. Continue working through your list day by day. As soon as you're ready, add one more thing. If you're not ready, continue at the same level until you are. If you slip back, decide to catch up again the next day. Or, if you've slipped for a few days, go back to the beginning. You're not in a race – but you can be sure of winning eventually, however fast or slowly you go.

I'm not suggesting for a minute that this is an instant cure for depression, but it is a way of regaining control.

- You have decided that taking certain actions will make you feel better than taking no action.
- You now know for a fact that, if you continue to progress through your list, you will feel better every day.
- You have the power to choose feeling good over feeling bad.

If you aren't able to move forward or you continue to feel overwhelmed, don't battle on alone. See your doctor, follow his or her advice and try again when you're feeling stronger.

Emphasise the positive

I found that checking off the positive things I had done for myself each day was such an inspiration that I threw in the things I had never let slip – like eating muesli for breakfast – to make myself feel even more virtuous!

15

YOU DON'T HAVE TO GET BACK TO NORMAL

- **You may feel depressed when you stop your treatment**
- **Create a new 'normal' to move forward to**
- **Living with the fear**

My treatment lasted for 34 weeks and, like everyone else who knew me, I expected to feel over the moon when it finished. I had heard that some people feel depressed when their treatment ends but dismissed that as seriously strange. It was only as my last dose of chemotherapy drew closer that I started understand how this could happen.

- Treatment can give you a sense of security. I certainly felt more protected from new cancers as long as I was having chemotherapy, even though I knew this wasn't necessarily the case.

- You may be worried that you haven't had enough treatment, or that it hasn't done everything it should. I had a niggling concern that my relatively symptom-free second course of chemotherapy meant it wasn't working properly.

- Ending your treatment means losing touch with people to whom you might feel very close. Your medical team may (and should) have been providing high levels of support and understanding. It can be easy to feel abandoned and alone.

Unlikely as it may sound, illness and treatment may have also had a positive role to play in your life.

- You may have enjoyed extra attention and care from your family and friends.

- You may have felt that your family finally appreciated you, and worry that they will soon go back to taking you for granted.

- You may have enjoyed the feeling of being removed from reality. Being ill can have a similar effect to being on holiday – it's a chance to put some of your worries on hold.

In my case, the thing I found most rewarding was feeling less pressured to perform in my job. I had an unassailable excuse – it's a hard man or woman who will complain about copy being a few hours late when the culprit is being treated for cancer. I also enjoyed being told how brave and strong I was, and knowing that people were more likely to be saying good things about me than bad things (yes, I'm paranoid!).

The reality is, while everyone is telling you how fabulous it will be to get back to normal, 'normal' may not that wonderful. You may not want to go back there at all.

As you can imagine, the last thing I would want to do is to go back to where I was before cancer. Back then I was the queen of the 'yes, but'. If anyone dared suggest that I change anything about my life I had a get-out for every occasion – 'yes, but I don't have enough money to do that', or 'yes, but I have four children - I don't have any time'.

If that's the case, this is a great moment to decide you're not going to. If you haven't already established your goals, do it now. Think about what you want your future to hold and plan to achieve it, and how much more health and happiness has to offer than illness and treatment.

Living with the fear

Cancer is a frightening illness and, unfortunately, the nature of cancer means there's unlikely to be a quick or specific end to the fear.

My first taste of the continuing fear came early.

Within days of my last chemotherapy treatment I developed a pain in my lower ribs.

At first I assumed it was a result of radiotherapy - perhaps even one of the spontaneous fractures I've been told can happen sometimes. Then I realised that the pain was below the treated area. Surely if this particular rib hadn't been weakened by radiotherapy I would remember an injury severe enough to crack a bone?

It was like déjà vu. I had the same sick feeling as when I first found the lump in my breast. One minute, I was the world's worst hypochondriac, next minute I was dying from a secondary tumour in the bone. I barely slept the night between having an x-ray and getting the result – that everything was fine.

I'm sure one of the hardest things facing people who have had cancer is finding a balance between panic and reasonable caution.

As members of the Cancer Club we have all lost a layer of protection that non-members take for granted – an intrinsic belief that 'it will never happen to me'. Of course we feel more vulnerable. We're allowed to.

I used to hope that the fear would recede over time and I'm glad to say it has. Of course I still have my moments but I'm not sure whether I have any more moments now than any other woman of my age. The difference is that I know more about cancer and I'm afraid of recurrence rather than diagnosis, so I suspect it affects the way I respond if something starts to worry me.

For instance, just a few weeks ago I became aware of a soapy taste in my mouth which was persistent enough to leave me feeling slightly nauseous. As soon as I realised it had been there for a while I put my hand on where I think my liver might be to see if it felt swollen – as if I'd know! Then I searched for 'soapy taste in mouth' on the Internet.

I hardly dared to look in case 'cancer in the liver' appeared in the same sentence because that, of course, was what I was afraid of. It didn't – but I still wasn't convinced. I started searching for 'symptoms of secondary liver cancer' and still couldn't find a connection. But I couldn't find an alternative explanation either, so the fear continued to nag away at the back of my mind. I gave myself a week before I would go to the doctor.

A couple of days later, I took a sip of tea just after putting on lip salve and I got an immediate and very strong taste of soap. I had been using a new brand and, yes, it tastes a bit soapy, but I hadn't put two and two together until the hot tea intensified the effect.

While I might not have been so focused in my research if I had never had cancer, the whole process made me realise that it had been months since I had felt moved to look up anything to do with advanced disease. Fear is no longer a big factor in my life. However, if the truth hadn't dawned within the week I allowed, I really would have told a doctor about it.

If you do find anything that concerns you – a lump or a pain, even a feeling that something's not quite right, don't be embarrassed about asking your doctor. If he or she isn't sympathetic, kind and quick to take appropriate action where it's needed, find one who is. You've been through a lot – this is the least you deserve.

Ongoing treatment

When I went to see my oncologist at the end of my Taxol treatment he recommended that I start a five-year course of Tamoxifen. I burst into tears. Yes, part of me was feeling insecure because my treatment had finished. But another part of me was relieved that I could start putting cancer behind me.

I also knew very little about Tamoxifen except that it had something to do with blocking oestrogen. Despite the fact that I had been perimenopausal at the time of my diagnosis and was now well and truly post menopausal, this scared the wits out of me. I had visions of shrivelling up like a walnut, ageing thirty years overnight and growing a luxuriant beard and moustache. Through my tears, I actually told my startled oncologist that I didn't want to turn into a dog-faced woman. He'd listened to all kinds of concerns in his time but his expression told me he'd never heard that one!

Of course I can see now that my reaction was all about being emotionally raw. When I calmed down we discussed the real pluses and minuses of Tamoxifen and I left feeling that it was probably a good thing. Once again I was lucky in terms of side effects – I had absolutely none, took it for five years and then, when I heard that the latest protocol was to follow this with five years of Arimidex, I didn't have a problem. Once again, I have had absolutely no side effects that I am aware of so far.

On the subject of side effects, I do find it fascinating that different people react so very differently to the same medication. There can be a fine line between those you feel you can manage and those which make your life unbearable. Always talk to your doctor – there may be alternatives that work better for you.

Please return this book
When you are finished
with it — Thanks -
(see inside front cover)

16

STAYING WELL
AFTER BREAST CANCER
- save $10

While I've touched on eating and exercise in this book, the sequel *STAYING WELL AFTER BREAST CANCER – A GENTLE GUIDE TO TAKING CARE OF THE BASICS* – goes a lot more deeply into the issues around emotional eating.

Evidence is mounting that maintaining a healthy weight and staying physically active are two of the most important things we can do to protect ourselves from getting breast cancer again. But managing your weight is never easy. When you're still reeling from the physical and emotional impact of a life-threatening disease, pressure to 'go on a diet' could feel like the final straw.

Personal experience has taught me that a healthy weight has nothing to do with willpower or deprivation. It's not about being 'on a diet' for a certain period of time. Rather, it's an integral part of a happier and more fulfilled life.

After breast cancer I learned to replace 'feel bad, diet, break diet, feel worse' with 'feel good, eat well, feel even better'. It's a gentle approach that I know can work and that, like feeling more positive, can be learned.

While the two books cover different topics they're based on the same principles and some information appears in both. I couldn't avoid this – much as I would love to, I can't assume that everyone has read both and either committed one to memory or keeps it handy enough to refer to!

Nevertheless, I'd hate anyone to feel short changed by this. That's why, if you would now like to read *STAYING WELL AFTER BREAST CANCER*, I'd like you to have it for $14.95 – a saving of $10 on the normal retail price of $24.95.

To take advantage of this offer, simply visit **www.doministuart.com** and write 'special offer' after your name on the order form.

"Staying Well After Breast Cancer is fantastic. I could not agree more with your whole outlook on this. I am tremendously impressed with the data on lifestyle, weight control, exercise, and reduction of relapse rates and push it very strongly now with all my patients."

Richard Kefford MB BS (Syd) PhD FRACP
Professor of Medicine at the University of Sydney
Chair of the Division of Medicine, Westmead Hospital, Sydney
Director of the Westmead Institute for Cancer Research

RECIPES

I don't pretend to be a chef or to be creating world-shattering new dishes – these are simply a few of the things I enjoyed throughout my treatment. I've tried to stick to dishes that are easy to prepare, are nutritious, can serve for more than one meal and can be as bland or tasty as you choose depending on how you feel.

PORRIDGE
Warming, nourishing and wonderfully bland, instant versions are also available.

Ingredients (one serving)
500 mil water or a mix of milk and water
I heaped tablespoon oats
Pinch of salt

Method
1. Bring the liquid to the boil.
2. Slowly pour in the oats, stirring all the time with a wooden spoon until the liquid has come back to the boil.
3. Add salt, reduce the heat, cover the pan and simmer very gently for 20-25 minutes, stirring frequently, until the porridge is thick but still able to be poured.
4. Serve hot with honey or raw sugar and a little extra milk if you like

MUESLI

We're told that it's good to eat a wide variety of foods, and that makes muesli a great way to start the day. You can buy excellent organic mueslis – I supplement mine with extra sunflower seeds, pumpkin seeds, pecan nuts and fruit. It's also easy to make your own and, that way, you can adjust the quantities to your own taste.

Starting with a base of rolled oats, simply add any or all of the following in the proportion you like best:

Flakes of rice or wheat or barley (toasted if you like)
Dried fruit – sultanas, apricots, peaches, apples, dates, mangoes
Nuts – almonds, pecans, brazil nuts, hazel nuts
Sunflower kernels
Pumpkin seeds
Oat bran
Linseed
Coconut

It's a good idea to toss the chopped, dried fruit pieces in oat bran before adding them to the mixture to stop them from sticking together. Use your fingers to make sure they're thoroughly coated.

You can serve your muesli with milk, soy milk or fruit juice and add any fresh fruit you fancy.

RATATOUILLE

Ingredients

1 tbsp oil
1 onion, chopped
2 cloves garlic, chopped
2 zucchini, sliced
1 green capsicum, chopped
1 medium eggplant, chopped
2 x 425g tins of tomatoes or 4 large, ripe, fresh tomatoes
A pinch of dried mixed herbs or a handful of fresh herbs

Method

1. Heat the oil and gently sauté the onion and garlic until soft.
2. Add the capsicum and zucchini and stir for a minute.
3. Add the eggplant, tomatoes and herbs.
4. Simmer for 45 minutes.

This is excellent with baked potatoes – just wash the potatoes, prick them with a fork and pop them in a preheated oven (about 180°C) as you start to cook the ratatouille.

VERSATILE SOUP

Soup is wonderful for eating in small quantities throughout the day when your appetite is a little jaded.

Simple Potato Soup was the only thing I could face after my first chemotherapy treatment but, if you don't feel nauseous, go straight past this recipe. Bland isn't the word!

Tasty Potato Soup is basis for any number of delicious vegetable soups – simply replace one or more potato with a similar weight of carrots, parsnips, sweet potato, leeks, cauliflower, broccoli or anything else you fancy.

SIMPLE POTATO SOUP

Ingredients
One onion
A tiny amount of oil
4 large potatoes, peeled and roughly chopped
A little salt if you like it

Method
1. Chop the onion finely and sauté it slowly in the smallest possible quantity of oil, or oil with a little water, until it's transparent.
2. Add the potatoes, enough water barely to cover them and salt if you're using it.
3. Bring to the boil and simmer until the potatoes are very tender.
4. Purée the soup in a blender or food processor.

TASTY POTATO SOUP

Ingredients
1 tbsp vegetable oil
One onion, chopped
3 or 4 cloves or garlic, chopped
4 large potatoes (or equivalent) roughly chopped
2 tsp Vegemite or Promite, or 2 vegetable stock cubes
500ml water
500ml milk or soy milk
Herbs – preferably fresh – such as parsley, oregano or sage
or thyme

Method
1. Heat the oil and gently sauté the onion and garlic until
   soft.
2. Stir in the chopped vegetables and stir well.
3. Add the water, Vegemite, Promite or stock cubes and
   herbs.
4. Simmer until the vegetables are very soft – about 30
   minutes.
5. Remove from the heat and purée in a food processor or
   blender until smooth.
6. Stir in the milk or soy milk and reheat without boiling.

To make the soup more tasty still, throw in a few
spices just before you add the vegetables and water and stir
over a low heat for a minute. ½ - 1 teaspoon each of ground
cumin, coriander and cardamom are good to start with. If
your mouth isn't too sore, add a teaspoon of ginger and a
pinch of chilli powder.

PASTA SAUCE

This tomato sauce is incredibly fast and easy to make and delicious on its own, especially if you use fresh tomatoes. For years I used canned tomatoes because I couldn't be bothered to peel fresh ones. Now I just leave the peel on – you don't notice it, and the flavour is so much nicer. While the sun dried tomatoes aren't essential, they really intensify the flavour. The sauce can be frozen, and it's easy to ring in the changes with a few extra ingredients.

Ingredients
1 tbsp oil
1 onion, chopped
2 cloves garlic, chopped
4 large, ripe tomatoes or 1 x 425g tin tomatoes
Juice of half a lemon, or a splash of red or white wine
3 or 4 sun dried tomatoes, drained and chopped (optional)
Fresh or dried herbs

Method
1. Gently sauté the onion and garlic in the oil until soft.
2. Add the tomatoes, herbs and lemon juice or wine.
3. Simmer for 15 minutes.
4. Serve with your favourite pasta and a salad.

Variations
Add any or all of the following:

- A handful of black olives
- Sliced mushrooms
- Chopped celery (sauté with the onions)
- Sliced zucchini or acorn squash
- ½ cup pine nuts, dry roasted in a non-stick pan

- Chopped capsicum
- A well-drained can of tuna
- Crumbled feta
- If your mouth's up to it, a chopped chilli (again, sauté with the onions) or a sprinkle of chilli flakes.

PESTO PRONTO!

Good quality pesto sauce is readily available in jars or from fresh food cabinets. Nothing could be faster than stirring it straight into hot pasta or gnocchi, which cooks in about two minutes flat. A great standby.

PIZZA

If you have a supply of ready-made pizza bases in the freezer you can whip up something that feels like a real meal in the time it takes to make a sandwich. Simply cover the base with tomato paste, a quality bottled pasta sauce or, to ring in the changes, pesto or olive tapenade. Add your choice of toppings, sprinkle on a little grated cheese and pop it into a hot oven until the cheese melts. Choose from:

- sliced vegetables – tomato, mushroom, red onion, capsicum, zucchini
- roasted vegetables – potato, sweet potato, pumpkin
- olives, capers, fresh herbs
- drained salmon or tuna
- anything else you like that's handy – have you seen what they put on gourmet pizzas these days? It is, however, best to avoid preserved meats like salami and ham.

VEGETABLE STEW

The number of vegetables involved makes this stew quite labour intensive, but it will last for three days in the fridge so it's a wise investment of time. It's very nutritious and easy to eat, and a great way to use up vegetables too.

Ingredients
1 tbsp oil
1 onion, chopped
2 cloves garlic, chopped
1 tbsp Vegemite or Promite, or two vegetable stock cubes
Vegetables – at least two of the following. Use them all if you like – and feel free to add anything else you fancy. Quantities are just a guide.

- 2-3 stalks celery, chopped
- 3 medium potatoes
- 2 large carrots, sliced
- 2 large parsnips, chopped
- 1 medium sweet potato, diced
- Swede, chopped
- Turnip, chopped
- ½ cauliflower broken into florets
- 1 cup peas, fresh or frozen
- 2 sliced zucchini
- 1 x 425g tin of beans, drained and rinsed – butter beans, kidney beans, mixed beans, soy beans or chick peas
- 1 tsp mixed dried herbs or a handful of chopped fresh herbs
- A bay leaf

Optional extras
- handful of cashew nuts
- ½ cup pearled barley

Method
1. Heat the oil and sauté the onion, celery and garlic until soft.
2. Turn up the heat and add the sliced carrots, parsnips and cauliflower. Stir until they're starting to brown.
3. Add potato, sweet potato, turnip, swede and herbs with enough water just to cover them, plus Vegemite, Promite or stock cubes and barley if you're using it.
4. Bring to boil and simmer for 15 minutes or until the vegetables and barley are cooked.
5. Add peas and zucchini.
6. Simmer for 5 minutes more.
7. Remove from heat and purée about one third of the stew in a blender. Return blended mixture to the pan.
8. Add beans and nuts, stir and serve with bread or toast.

ROASTED VEGETABLES

Simply toss cut-up potato, sweet potato, parsnip and pumpkin with a little olive oil, place them in a single layer on a baking tray and sprinkle with a little sea salt.

If you have fresh rosemary, lay a couple of sprigs over the vegetables, then bake them in the over for about 45 minutes at 180°C.

SPICY POTATOES

In a bowl, mix together 1 tablespoon olive oil, 1 teaspoon each of ground cumin, coriander and cardamom, plus a little ground ginger and chilli if your mouth isn't too sore. Wash and dice 4 medium potatoes, dry them on a cloth then tip them into the oil and spices and stir until they're all well coated. Arrange them in a single layer on a baking tray and cook them at 180°C for about 45 minutes.

COOL CURRY

Even if your mouth is sore you can enjoy tasty, Indian-inspired meals. Use individual spices rather than a ready-made curry powder and you have the option of leaving out the chilli and ginger, so you can enjoy the flavour without the heat. This recipe is delicious, and a great way of transforming left-over cooked vegetables.

Ingredients
1 tbsp oil
1 tsp black mustard seeds
1 tbsp cumin seeds
Chopped chilli, or pinch chilli powder (optional)
1 cup cooked vegetables (spinach, potatoes and peas are particularly good)

Method
1. Heat the oil and fry the mustard seeds until they start to pop
2. Add the cumin seeds and stir for one minute
3. Add the vegetables and stir until heated through.
4. Serve with rice or Indian bread.

DHAL

Ingredients

1 cup red lentils, rinsed well
3cm fresh ginger, sliced
1 cinnamon stick
2 tbsp oil
1 large onion, finely chopped
2 cloves garlic, crushed
2 tsp turmeric
1 tsp cumin
1/2 tsp garam marsala
Up to ½ tsp chilli flakes (optional)
English spinach (optional)
2 tbsp lemon juice
Salt to taste
Torn coriander leaves to taste

Method

1. Place lentils, ginger and cinnamon in a large saucepan with 3 cups of cold water. Bring to the boil, reduce the heat to medium and simmer, stirring occasionally, for 10-12 minutes. Remove and discard the spices.
2. Fry the onion and garlic over a medium heat until soft.
3. Stir in the garlic, turmeric, cumin, garam marsala and chilli flakes and fry gently for a minute or so.
4. Add the lentils and lemon juice, mix well and cook for a few minutes longer, stirring continuously.
5. If you're using spinach, add it now and stir it through until it wilts.
6. Sprinkle with the coriander leaves just before serving.
7. Serve hot with naan bread or rice.

FRUIT CRUMBLE

This 'dessert' is so nutritious that I sometimes have it as a main meal!

Ingredients

4 medium apples
½ cup water
4 tbsp rolled oats
1 tbsp plain flour – preferably wholemeal
1 tbsp desiccated coconut
2 tbsp chopped almonds, pecans or walnuts
1 tbsp sunflower seeds
1 tbsp tahini (the lighter, hulled variety of sesame paste works best)
1 tbsp honey

Method

1. Peel and slice the apples into a saucepan. Add the water, bring to the boil and simmer until apples are tender.
2. Combine the remaining ingredients in a bowl. It's best to use your hands for this.
3. Lightly grease a small pie dish and tip in the fruit and juice
4. Smooth the crumble mix over the top and press down lightly.
5. Cook in a preheated oven at 200°C for about 15 minutes, until the top is starting to brown.
6. Serve hot or cold, alone or with custard, cream or ice cream for a treat!

Variations

You can use just about any fruit in season, either alone or mixed with some apple. Try rhubarb (add a little extra honey when you're cooking it), apricots, peaches, plums and berries.

SMOOTHIES

Frozen Berry Smoothie
Ingredients
1 cup low fat yoghurt
1/2 cup milk, skim milk or soy milk
1/2 cup of frozen berries or any frozen fresh fruit

Banana Smoothie
Ingredients
1peeled banana, sliced
2 tbsp natural yoghurt
200ml milk
1 tsp honey
1 tbsp wheat germ (optional)
60ml 1/4 cup orange juice
Method for both
Simply whiz all the ingredients together in a blender until they're smooth and creamy.

INDEX